Acupuncture

ACUPUNCTURE

A Viable
Medical Alternative

MARIE CARGILL

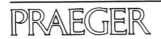

Westport, Connecticut
London

While the advice and information in this book are believed to be true and accurate at the date of going to press, neither the author nor the publisher can accept any legal responsibility for any errors or omissions that may be made. The publisher makes no warranty, express or implied, with respect to the matter contained herein. Readers are encouraged to confirm the information in this volume with other sources.

Library of Congress Cataloging-in-Publication Data

Cargill, Marie.
    Acupuncture : a viable medical alternative / Marie Cargill.
        p.   cm.
    Includes bibliographical references and index.
    ISBN 0–275–94881–1 (pbk.)
        1. Acupuncture—Popular works.   I. Title.
    RM184.C37   1994
    615.8'92—dc20   94–12069

British Library Cataloguing in Publication Data is available.

Library of Congress Catalog Card Number: 94–12069
ISBN: 0–275–94881–1 (pbk.)

First published in 1994

Praeger Publishers, 88 Post Road West, Westport, CT 06881
An imprint of Greenwood Publishing Group, Inc.

Printed in the United States of America

∞™

The paper used in this book complies with the
Permanent Paper Standard issued by the National
Information Standards Organization (Z39.48–1984).

10 9 8 7 6 5 4

To my mother, Rose Deraedt

An important scientific innovation rarely makes its way by gradually winning over and converting its opponents; it rarely happens that Saul becomes Paul. What does happen is that its opponents gradually die out and that the growing generation is familiarized with the idea from the beginning.

Max Planck

CONTENTS

Part 3   Acupuncture in the United States

Illustrations and photographs follow Chapter 9.

PREFACE

Great numbers of Americans are choosing alternatives to conventional medical care. Even so, most people are aware of only a few of the many ways acupuncture can restore and maintain health. Many people know that acupuncture can relieve pain, and some know that it can help curb addiction to alcohol, drugs, cigarettes, and food. But this is the limit of general awareness of acupuncture in this country. This book attempts to fill this gap and to present a rounded introduction to the field of acupuncture. It is impossible to provide in one book an overview of a body of knowledge and medical practice that is every bit as extensive as that of Western medicine. I must, therefore, be selective. The Introduction and first four chapters will give you a bit of background information and will describe some of the central concepts of acupuncture. I will discuss theories that underlay the practice of acupuncture, and I will also describe recent scientific attempts to explain how and why acupuncture works.

This work will involve brief excursions into neurology, anatomy, and brain chemistry. I will show you the tools we practitioners use, explain how a diagnosis is made, and discuss some actual cases I have treated.

Chapters 5 through 16 cover the special areas in which acupuncture has proven effective: pain management, anesthesiology, brain disease, and injuries. I will talk about pediatrics, gynecology, internal medicine, and cancer. In discussing these and other topics, I will draw on research from around the world. I will also provide information from clinical literature and relate case histories from my own practice.

In the two concluding chapters, I will tell you about the current scientific and legal status of acupuncture in the United States. I will discuss the preventive advantages of using acupuncture as an alternative treatment and demonstrate its cost-effectiveness. I will then advise you how to go about adding acupuncture to your general health management program.

Throughout this book I have tried to avoid using technical jargon and to explain terms and specialized vocabulary as they appear. At the end of each chapter I have included sources for the material covered. These books and articles can serve as a guide to further reading. A bibliography provides a list of readily available works that will allow the interested reader to explore in greater detail all the topics I've introduced. An appendix lists associations that can help you select your own acupuncturist.

ACKNOWLEDGMENTS

I am indebted to the following people for their support, suggestions and editing through the years of putting this manuscript together: Neils Braroe, Patrick Cournil, Edye Cox, Nick Dussault, Bill Grealish, Kathy Hennessey, Larry Hitt, Alice Koller, Rhea Moquin, Carol Page, Josephine Roccuzzo and Donna Wood. My thanks to my agent, Joseph S. Ajlouny. I also acknowledge a great debt to all my patients for sharing their thoughts, feelings, and experiences on the process of acupuncture.

Part 1

BASICS

Introduction

MY PATH TO ACUPUNCTURE

I am a practitioner of Oriental medicine. In China, I would be called "Doctor Cargill"; in the United States I am not permitted to use that title. When I fulfilled the requirements for being licensed to practice acupuncture in Massachusetts, I agreed not to call myself "doctor." It seems a small matter, but it reflects a view held by many Americans that only practitioners of Western medicine are worthy of the name. Such preconceptions help to keep Americans unaware that acupuncture, in combination with herbal medicine, can restore and maintain health. If these medical resources were widely available, patients and their insurance companies would no longer have to spend vast sums of money for hospitals, surgery, and medication. Acupuncture can alleviate prolonged pain, discomfort, and anxiety, and end severe dependence on a medical system so huge and impersonal that each patient feels like a forgotten cog in a machine.

I'm an American, born and reared in the United States. It may seem odd that I choose to practice another country's medicine. I might have taken the same path that hundreds of American women take every year and simply have entered medical school. I will tell you why I chose not to.

Initially, I had no leaning toward medicine. In high school I wasn't drawn to biology, chemistry, or the "hard sciences." I was an artist: I wanted to draw, paint, and work with color. After receiving my bachelor's degree from the Massachusetts College of Art, I taught for two years at the elementary level in a lovely town in upstate New York. I decided to continue my studies and returned to Boston, where I received a Master of Fine Arts degree from Boston University. Then, for nearly four years I had my own studio, designing fabrics and making prints. Although I have an artist's hand and eye, I do not have a head for business, so I closed my studio and looked for another teaching job. For a year I was a Master Teacher in a Head Start program. Longing more for expanded art experience than for education, I spent the next year traveling around the world. I went from Japan, the Philippines, and India to Egypt, Greece, and Italy.

I traveled over the Alps to Switzerland, Germany, France and Holland, and I crossed the channel to England and Scotland before coming home. I brought back luggage filled with fabrics, jewelry, and whatever else of beauty had caught my eye in these countries. And then I settled down. For the next twelve years I was a public school system arts administrator, responsible for nurturing the artistic lives of an entire town's citizenry, from kindergarten through adult continuing education.

During my tenth year in this occupation, my father developed a prostate problem. His urinary tract became obstructed, and, because of urine backup, toxicity was an imminent danger. My father was in great discomfort. To restore his health, he agreed to undergo the surgery that his doctors had been urging. The operation was successful in clearing up the prostate problem, but it destroyed the man who had been my father. Immediately after regaining consciousness, he had no idea who he was or why he was in the hospital. He did not recognize us, his wife and his daughter. When he was strong enough to walk, he would wander aimlessly through hospital corridors. One day he dressed himself and left. For two hours, we were in complete panic until he was found again.

From the time of his surgery onward, his actions became bizarre: he seemed to have become a disoriented spirit trapped in a body, unconnected to those who loved him.

His doctors persuaded my mother and me that his depression and memory loss would best be evaluated in a psychiatric hospital, so we consented to signing admission papers. Without consulting us, new doctors subjected him to electroconvulsive shock therapy (ECT). My father endured severe shock treatments before we learned what was being done. My mother was outraged and protested to the hospital administrator, who at first evaded her telephone calls. When she finally confronted officials in person, they refused to be responsible in any way for the actions of their staff physicians. We promptly consulted a lawyer, who sent a strong letter to the Massachusetts Board of Medical Ethics. Only then was ECT suspended, and my father's doctors reluctantly agreed to explain to us their diagnosis of his problems and treatment plan they were considering.

With no time to recover from the ECT, his doctors pushed him into the next treatment stage: the mind-altering drugs Haldol and Thorazine.

My father developed several of the worst possible adverse reactions to psychotropic drugs and disappeared into the shadows of life. He was alive, but so remote that he could not talk, eat, walk, think, or behave as one would expect in a 66-year-old.

We won his release from the hospital. My mother undertook the arduous job of caring for him much as she had cared for me when I was a small child, feeding him, meeting his basic needs for cleanliness, never leaving him alone. He lived for two more years. When he died we were both bitter, angry, and disillusioned with the medical system that had caused this tragedy.

We did not know then that there were alternative treatments, and so we returned to the same medical system when my exhausted mother fell ill a few months later. The severe and inextricable stress of the preceding years had made some sort of illness predictable. First, she experienced pain in her chest and upper back. The pain led to further complications: loss of appetite, insomnia, and depression. She began a merry-go-round of consultations with a series of specialists. Each had a different diagnosis; each had a different treatment plan.

Each looked on her as a piece of mechanical equipment they could tinker with. Doctors lost interest in her when their tinkering did no good, and they dismissed her as if she caused them problems by presenting them with symptoms they could not relieve. Of course, they intimated that her problems were "in her head" and not real.

This coming and going to doctors lasted several months, while she continued to suffer pain. We often wondered whether there might be some alternative to the useless attention she'd been receiving. One day a friend phoned and listened to my mother's despair and grief. She came to our house and scooped up my mother and took her to a new doctor—a doctor of Oriental medicine. From her first treatment, her life started to turn around.

My mother was in her early 60s at the time, and her pain was severe. It had lasted long enough to be considered chronic. The series of acupuncture treatments lasted several months. Gradually and steadily, the pain subsided. She ate and slept well again, and her depression lifted. She recovered fully.

I watched her progress with amazement and gratitude. I could not help comparing it to the medical fiasco that deprived my father of his mind and his spirit, and finally took his life. In only a few months, I made some important decisions. I left my secure and safe education job of thirteen years, applied and was accepted into the only acupuncture teaching institute in the New England area, The New England School of Acupuncture.

My training was both intensive and extensive. I had classroom courses in theory, pathology, and diagnosis, point location, and needle practice. My class studied different schools of acupuncture—Korean, Japanese, and Chinese. We constantly reviewed case studies and the results of clinical research. We were apprenticed in clinics where the student trained under and assisted a different practicing acupuncturist each semester. I interned at the Lemuel Shattuck Hospital in Boston, where acupuncture was integrated with therapeutic massage, psychological counseling, physiotherapy, art and movement therapy, nutrition, and, of course, Western medicine. At the New England School of Acupuncture we also had courses in anatomy and physiology. In addition, we were given overviews of medical specialties and some training in pharmacology.

After I completed the three-year course of study in acupuncture, I elected to continue studying herbal medicine, a decision that added three more years of part-time study to my training. In the United States, acupuncture and herbal medicine are separate fields; one does not have to take both courses of study to qualify for licensing as an acupuncturist.

At the New England School of Acupuncture, the first year of the herbal medicine course involved learning each traditional herb, its modes of preparation, and the correct administration for specific ailments. I learned the properties of each herbal medicine and its application to specific complaints, whether acute or chronic. The second year continued with herbal prescriptions and the nearly unlimited possible combinations of herbal substances. In my last year I was given intensive instruction in the applications of herbal prescriptions in internal medicine.

Throughout my education, I chose to apprentice myself to the

Boston acupuncturist who cured my mother, Dr.YunWon Suh. I worked with him weekly while attending regular classes.

Eleven years ago, I opened my own practice. I have continued to practice acupuncture despite the high level of frustration I feel dealing with a rigid and unresponsive Western medical bureaucracy. As my knowledge of Traditional Chinese Medicine deepens and broadens, I have added teaching and research to my clinical practice. I regularly give lectures and workshops to interested lay audiences. I now cannot imagine a life without herbal remedies and acupuncture, whether administering them or receiving them myself. My mother, by the way, is still doing well at 80.

Chapter 1

WHAT IS ACUPUNCTURE?

The medical practice you will read about in this book is unique. It is relatively new in the United States, constituting a revolutionary approach to health care. It can make you feel as healthy and vital as you have always wanted to be. Yet it is a medicine with a history thousands of years old and has enriched the lives of millions of people. Often, in just a few simple treatments, your health problems can be reversed completely, freeing you from disease and pain. Acupuncture will also help ensure against relapse or developing future illnesses.

Acupuncture is now widely practiced in this country, although it has not yet entered the medical mainstream of clinics, hospitals, and insurance plans. It has already helped hundreds of thousands of Americans.

Western and Eastern medicine have different focuses. A conventional Western doctor looks at a patient's body through the lens of disease theory. He records symptoms according to a rigidly defined set of tangible categories. He sets about to isolate the disease and control it by destroying the agents that cause it. His techniques invade the body by either cutting into it or by introducing powerful chemicals into it.

A doctor trained in Traditional Chinese Medicine (TCM) regards the same patient in a more holistic manner, considering all of his or her body systems, mental states, and lifestyle. She asks about the patient's environment and his or her relationship to it. In making a diagnosis, she looks for a pattern of disharmony that emerges from all these observations, and then she proceeds to restore health by cultivating natural harmony. The contrast in Eastern and Western approaches can be illustrated by comparing ways of treating the common ulcer.

One of my professors, Dr. Ted Kaptchuk, is fond of using this example. Confronted with six patients suffering with stomach pain, a Western physician subjects each of them to an endoscopy, an upper gastrointestinal X-ray test that is costly and time consuming, involves several specialists and technicians, and is quite uncomfortable for the patient. If the results are positive, a diagnosis of peptic ulcer is made. Usually, only one treatment is prescribed: drugs and dietary changes. Surgery may be performed in very severe cases. The outcome is usually problematic: some patients improve only to have a recurrence years later; other patients never improve.

Now, if the same six people are sent to a Traditional Chinese Medical doctor, their experience and treatment will be radically different. They will be listened to and asked numerous, seemingly "irrelevant" questions. They will be palpated (their bodies touched and examined) and have their pulses taken. The doctor will pay special attention to their tongues: much information about a person's health can be gleaned from the tongue. Gradually, six different pictures of disharmony will emerge, each calling for a different set of measures.

The first patient is robust with a ruddy complexion and seems to have a strong personality. He complains of frequent constipation and dark urine. The doctor finds that his stomach pain increases when a certain place is touched and decreases when cold compresses are applied.

The second patient is thin. His skin lacks luster. He is nervous. He says that he is always thirsty and that he has sweaty palms and night sweats. He suffers from insomnia. He likens his pain to the throb of a toothache.

Eating always brings temporary relief to the third patient. He reports that he is always sleepy, sweats spontaneously, and gets up often during the night to urinate. He prefers cold weather. He is pale and timid.

The fourth patient describes sharp, stabbing pain accompanied by sour belching. She has frequent headaches. She describes herself as moody and says that emotional upset brings on pain that can sometimes be lessened by massage.

Patient number five has severe, stabbing pain that sometimes travels from her stomach to her back. She is overweight, with a pale face and shiny skin. She complains that her stools are often loose. Heat applications sometimes help reduce the pain.

The sixth patient has cramping pain. The pain is much worse just after eating; at this time he cannot stand being touched. He vomits blood at times and has very dark stools. He is thin with a dull, dark complexion.

After acupuncture treatment, the practitioner of Chinese Medicine will not only have cured all six patients of the ailments lumped together as "ulcers," but he will have relieved most of their other symptoms as well. Gone will be constipation, belching, headaches, painful menstrual periods, vomiting, hemorrhaging, night sweats, thirst and frequent urination, diarrhea, and mood swings.

These were real patients who underwent acupuncture treatment for an average of two months, as part of a large study on ulcers conducted in China. Throughout treatment they were given no drugs, nor was their diet restricted. Each patient was given special care tailored to his or her condition. This is the significant point: no two patients required the same treatment plan. When the results were evaluated using Western diagnostic techniques, fifty-three (83%) of the patients had recovered completely. Seven patients (11%) showed significant improvement, and two (3%) showed moderate improvement. Only two patients (3%) registered no progress at all. In other words, about 95 percent of the patients were either cured completely or showed varying degrees of improvement—without drugs and after only two short months of needling sessions.

How is this possible? In the following pages I will describe how Chinese Medicine approaches the person as a whole, unique individual rather than as the focus of an isolated disease. The Traditional Chinese Medicine (TMC) practitioner uses her skills and knowledge to restore the patient's body systems to harmony. In fact, maintaining this balance has come to be a kind of preventive medicine in China.

The Chinese word for medicine derives from three ancient ideograms or thought-pictures: alcohol stored in a bottle, an arrowhead kept in a box, and a hand grasping a weapon. The arrowhead is thought to represent the needle used to activate parts of the body. The Chinese word for acupuncture means "to wound with gold," and acupuncture needles found in the tomb of physician Liu Sheng, who died about 100 B.C., are made of gold. In clinics today, practitioners use stainless steel needles that are not much larger in diameter than a strand of thick hair. Physicians discovered that if they placed a needle just under the skin at certain points on the human body, predictable changes occurred. These points became the inventory of acupuncture points, and they lined themselves into pathways. With training, a practitioner could locate any desired point, needle it, and bring about desired change.

Chinese scientists discovered that the pathways not only traced themselves on the surface, but also interpenetrated all the layers of the body—the skin, muscles, tissues, organs, and bones. Such a system of multiple, intricate channels, weaving into and out of one another, can be thought of as a three-dimensional electrical circuit, like that in a house. Through this circuitry, a life force analogous to electricity travels with a speed that can be slowed down, increased, or stopped at many points along the way.

Present-day practitioners of acupuncture have modern as well as ancient circuit maps of points and channels. An example is the "Lung channel" that goes up the arm and over the chest. It has a definite route and can be needled at specific points to treat such maladies as congested sinuses, hacking cough, excessive perspiration, and constipation. Its points can be used to treat diseases of the lung and chest area. In making a diagnosis, the acupuncturist chooses exactly which point to needle, and she identifies these points by measuring, feeling with her fingers, and noting surface temperature changes, numbness, tingling, discolorations, and swelling along the channel route.

Acupuncture was exported from China and used extensively in Korea and Japan. In the seventeenth century, it was brought to Europe. The first work on acupuncture in a European language was by a Jesuit priest in 1671. France embraced acupuncture, and many of its distinguished physicians advocated the use of acupuncture in human and animal care. The Canadian physician Sir William Osler exported it across the Atlantic Ocean in the 1800's. He and his colleagues considered acupuncture to be extraordinarily effective for lumbago—low back pain.

In China, however, acupuncture very nearly died out. As China struggled to become modern, Western medicine was avidly embraced. After the founding of the People's Republic of China, the leaders of the revolution were convinced of its worth when they saw that it saved the lives of thousands of men, women, and animals during the Long March. And because Chinese leaders wanted to distance themselves ideologically from the West, acupuncture had the additional appeal of being homegrown.

Since 1949, thousand of books and articles have been published in China on acupuncture and herbal pharmacology. Practitioners have been trained at many levels, from barefoot rural doctors and veterinarians to anesthetists working in modern urban hospitals.

Today in China, acupuncture is seen as an integral field of medicine with limitless boundaries. Recent discoveries and new techniques have combined with classic acupuncture. New technologies, such as electroacupuncture and the use of lasers have been developed. Every graduate of modern medical schools has had both theoretical and clinical experience with Traditional Chinese Medicine, and students who specialize in clinical practice must take courses in Western medicine. Eastern and Western medicines have been successfully combined in operating rooms, clinics, and hospitals.

Japanese practitioners are now using acupuncture to treat many common ailments, and they have had spectacular results in treating serious disorders that have been stubbornly resistant to Western science. They report cures for some forms of deafness and blindness, both inherited and acquired. Paralyzed patients have walked again with acupuncture therapy. Acupuncture is also practiced in Africa, Europe, Southeast Asia, and in Middle East countries such as Israel and Egypt. It has become required study in many medical and dental schools, particularly in Scandinavia and Russia, and it has reduced the costs of health care where it has been adopted.

Western physicians have been reluctant to accept acupuncture, often because of a lack of knowledge about the medicine. Much of what we know in the United States comes from research in Europe and elsewhere. In this country the emphasis has been on how needling affects the nervous system and alleviates pain. Little study has been done on how acupuncture modifies blood chemistry, glandular secretions, and cellular fluids.

Like any field of medicine, acupuncture has its advantages, disadvantages, and limitations. The chief advantage is its value as an alternative to surgery and drugs in curing disease. Drugs and the trauma of surgery have grave side effects that can often make the cure worse than the cause. Because of its simplicity, acupuncture is also inexpensive; this makes it an attractive component of preventive medicine. A general disadvantage is that it takes time to work and requires patient commitment. An urgent, life-threatening situation can be best managed by Western technology. I must qualify this statement by adding that acupuncture is useful when it precedes major surgery and that it is appropriate in the earliest stages of the postsurgical healing process.

Acupuncture works for nine out of ten people. When it fails, the reasons can only be guessed at. The limitations of acupuncture are generally person-specific and cannot be established until needling has been tried and failed. Most often, it is likely that failure occurred because not enough time was allowed to complete a course of treatment, or patients may have taken drugs that have a cumulative blocking effect on acupuncture.

For the 90 percent of us who respond positively to acupuncture, the results are marvelous. If you are ill, if you suffer from any chronic degenerative disorder, then you should consider acupuncture. If you are basically healthy, and yet are bothered by vague, seemingly unrelated symptoms that come and go unaccountably, then you too are a candidate for acupuncture. And if you are fit and free from all disease, then acupuncture can play an important role in maintaining your energy level and keeping you vital for the rest of your life.

Let's begin with a case history that well illustrates some of the special aspects of Traditional Chinese Medicine. Elsa is a wife and mother in her mid-fifties. She is intent on maintaining her precious health and in caring for others. Her disease was not rare or exotic, even though it was elusive and puzzling to her and her doctors. She was so constantly ill that she could scarcely get through a day.

By the time Elsa came to see me, she had endured years of poor health. When we first sat and talked, she reminded me that she had called and arranged an appointment months before, but at the last minute had canceled. She suspected that acupuncture couldn't do anything for her because all the other cures she'd tried over the years had failed. Like many patients who come for the first consultation, she brought detailed notes to discuss and the results of blood and urine tests she'd had the previous three or four years. She had listed an array of vitamins and dietary supplements she was currently taking.

Elsa was convinced she had chronic fatigue syndrome (CFS). She had a checklist from a support group of CFS sufferers, pointing out that she had 70 percent of the symptoms. But, she went on, she had never been positively diagnosed with CFS because no sign had shown up in her blood tests. Now, she wanted to know, how could acupuncture help this real but unidentified affliction?

I said, "Let's back up and start with some questions. What would you call your main, most pervasive complaint?"

"I can't concentrate," she said. "That's the main thing. Second, I am very tired all of the time. I get stuck. I go over and over what I need to do, and even then I can't remember what I just thought about."

Now, even though the inability to think well and remember can be a part of CFS, this symptom is far from unique to it. We needed much more information. I asked her if she had any viral or flu-like symptoms.

"Yes. I often have sore throats and swollen glands. Not outright flues or colds, just on the edge of them."

"Do you have a cough or other chest problems?"

"No, no cough, but I do feel my heart beat. I wake every night about 3:00 a.m. and stay awake a couple of hours. I can fall back to a light sleep most of the time. When I can't, I just read or meditate or pray."

"Do you have digestive problems?"

"Terrible ones. My stomach hurts. I belch and break wind. I have heartburn and awful diarrhea. On some occasions I have lost complete control of my bowels. It is so embarrassing. Other times I am the opposite—constipated. I am nauseated a lot. I have hemorrhoids and bladder incontinence. Every part of the whole system is a complete mess."

I asked her to tell me about her menstrual cycle.

"I'm still menstruating, even at my age. My periods are very heavy and I get irritable and bloated. Plus, I crave sweets! Then I get depressed; it's a very unhappy few days every month." Elsa described mood swings that frequently assailed her. "I can best describe it by saying that I become very difficult to be with for no reason I can discover."

"You said you can't concentrate. Tell me about that."

"That is probably the most frightening part of whatever it is I have. I have no attention span. I cannot do simple chores or carry out step-by-step procedures like following a recipe. I get so frustrated. I can't remember where I am in the recipe or even what chore I'm supposed to be doing. I walk across the room and forget why when I get to the other side. The most scary thing that happened recently was that I left the house with a pot of soup going on the kitchen stove. I could have burned the house down with our dog in it. That would have made me completely crazy."

"What about fatigue," I asked. "Is this after exercise or just light exertion?"

Elsa said gravely, "I want you to realize that, first of all, I have not felt normal energy for years. I have no strength to do more than light housework. I have to push myself. There are times in the day when I just want to put my head down and sleep. But I know that if I do, I won't feel any better when I wake up. I have headaches, sometimes really severe. They go up the back of my head and all the way to the front of my eyes. I see flashing lights, and I can't tolerate bright lights. My hands and fingers are sometimes numb. Sometimes I am lightheaded and spacey. It's hard to describe; it's like I can't find the right words to say anything, or make my tongue say it right if I can."

I asked her to tell me any other problems she had, no matter how vague or seemingly unconnected. Elsa was well prepared with her list. She said that she had night sweats. She had cold hands and cold feet, muscle aches, and occasional rashes. She had periodic weight gain and hair loss.

Elsa sat back, blew her nose, and dabbed her eyes. "I've covered everything, I think." She had a challenging manner, and said, "Have you ever dealt with anyone as badly messed up as me?"

I explained to her that I had had patients very badly off, but not in exactly the same ways. This is because every person is unique; nobody's system is exactly like that of any other. If a person is going to be "messed-up," it will happen in her or his special messed-up way. I told her that the tools I work with, acupuncture and herbs, can help to turn many of these problems around. She should not expect complete, instant recovery, however. We would have to work at restoring her health. I asked if she could tolerate feeling poorly a while longer until my methods began to take hold.

Elsa had listened intently and understood that her journey would be long, perhaps frustrating at times, but there was an excellent possiblility of turning her life around if we persevered.

"All right. Let's start," she said.

From that meeting on, Elsa became my patient, coming for acupuncture twice a week and taking herbal medicines faithfully every day. We very carefully monitored her body's responses. Our determination paid off. I believed she had a thyroid problem and an autonomic system out of control, even though blood tests showed her to be in the normal range of functioning according to the criteria of Western medicine, but I felt we could turn her case around. As I started to treat her with Traditional Chinese Medical techniques appropriate to this diagnosis, Elsa showed improvement. My goal was to build up her energy level and to shift energy from some parts of her body to others. I worked to support her basic kidney and spleen energy—as it is understood in Traditional Chinese Medicine— and thereby to stimulate the functioning of her thyroid, pituitary, thymus, adrenal, and pancreatic systems.

Not every symptom cleared up at the same rate, but after six months of treatments, she was well on her way to recovery.

We agreed to cease biweekly treatments for a while to let her body continue its healing process. She happily reported to me that she felt "about 80 percent better." After a four-month hiatus, we resumed treatments. She continued to improve and has not slipped back into any of the old patterns of discomfort. We devised an ongoing treatment plan consisting of herbs and as maintenance and preventive treatment, instituted an acupuncture treatment every two months.

Elsa is, quite literally, a new woman. Her vitality and good humor have returned, and she now embraces life and all it has to offer. Her family life has begun to bring the rewards and pleasures she had always longed to experience. She is enthusiastically making plans for a small business venture.

Elsa was correct in believing that her persistent complex of disabling symptoms was unique. By recognizing relationships of symptoms and applying Chinese medicine theory, we were able to restore her to a condition of wholeness and balance.

REFERENCES

For more detailed information on Western and Chinese Medical correspondences, consult Ted J. Kaptchuk's *The Web That Has No Weaver* (1983). Two excellent sources of the history of Traditional Chinese Medicine are Yoshiaki Omura, *Acupuncture Medicine* (1982) and Paul U. Unschuld's *Forgotten Traditions of Ancient Chinese Medicine* (1990).

Chapter 2

A VISIT TO AN ACUPUNCTURIST

"Acupuncture in the hands of a skilled practitioner is considerably more complicated than much of modern mechanical practice," writes Rick Carlson in his book *The End of Medicine*. He explains that "an acupuncturist must possess a finely calibrated skill to read a patient's body. Knowledge of 365 acupuncture points and a sensitivity to some 12 different bodily pulses, or meridians, each with 27 gradations, is required."[1] The practitioner can locate hundreds of acupuncture points. She or she has cultivated sensitivity to the touch of a dozen energy levels along the surface of the body. What this means to the patient is that this one medical system can affect all the parts of your body. In the following description of a typical first visit by a new patient, you can begin to understand how we make a diagnosis and draw up a treatment plan.

Rosemarie has made an appointment to seek help with her hypertension, or high blood pressure. I've told her to allow an hour for this first visit because I will need to gather detailed information about her condition before I can determine the best strategy. She tells me that she was diagnosed several years ago with hypertension and has been taking medication ever since. So far, it hasn't helped: her blood pressure keeps rising. Her doctor has switched her from one drug to another with no improvement and has now suggested increasing the dosages. Rosemarie says that she is tired of taking drugs that don't work.

Now it is my turn. I ask routine questions about her medical history and learn that she has a low energy level, urinates frequently, has trouble sleeping, and frequently feels stress in her daily life. I probe for clues to her total health that might have gone unnoticed. Habits of eating, drinking, and elimination are important to my diagnosis. I inquire about illnesses or accidents in her past, whether she has had surgery, and what medications she has used over the years.

I ask if any of her complaints are worse at some specific point in the day and if they vary with the weather or season. I ask her to describe any aches or pains in detail. I want to know if her pain is localized or if it travels. Is it relieved by warmth or pressure? Is her discomfort aggravated by cold or exertion? We talk about all her body systems: circulation, respiration, digestion, elimination, and menstruation. We cover her sleeping and eating habits, her states of mind. After an hour together, I have begun to acquire a picture of her as a whole person, including how she functions at her best, not just when ill and in need of medical care.

The next step is a physical examination. I gently probe the abdominal area and examine her ears for any unusual signs. I give special attention to her tongue, noting its color, shape, size, and coatings. Then I take various pulses along the wrist to confirm the diagnosis I've already begun to formulate.

Western doctors are interested in just one pulse and usually only its frequency. We in Oriental medicine get information from both wrists. We position our fingers on three places on each side, and we use three different amounts of pressure at three different depths for each position. There are eighteen of these pulses and each has twenty-nine possible telltale characteristics. Every one of them gives us data on the internal workings of the patient's body—its balanced harmony or disharmony.

Now I am ready to present a treatment plan to Rosemarie; I tell her exactly what I am going to do with my needles. I describe to her how the needling will feel and what she can expect during and right after the treatment and over time in the course of future sessions. I assure her that the needle doesn't hurt going in. Acupuncture needles, as I have said, are only about as thick as a human hair, not like sewing needles or the thick needles Western doctors use to draw blood or inject medicine. My needles are positioned just under the skin, at various points on her body. At most, she will feel a very slight stinging sensation.

Insertion is done very quickly, with a steady hand movement or by aiming needles through a small tube. First-time patients, waiting anxiously for me to begin, are frequently surprised when I tell them that the needle is already in place. They will sit up and check to see if I'm telling the truth. Then they relax and begin to enjoy the session. Once the needle is inserted, I may manipulate it by rotating it. This, too, is usually painless.

The needles, I assure her, are completely sterile. An acupuncturist uses either disposable, presterilized, stainless steel needles that come blister-wrapped, or reusable sterilized ones. The latter are soaked after each use in an antiseptic solution and are carefully checked for nicks or rough edges. They are sterilized using standard equipment prescribed by hospitals and the Bureau of Disease Control. I always use disposable needles, and a patient can ask any acupuncturist to do likewise.

In Rosemarie's case, I have determined that needles will be placed at several points on the front of her body and at other points on her back. These points are chosen to bring about predictable changes in her overall body disharmony. When I place the needles in the front, she tells me that she feels a slight tingling. After about twenty minutes, we repeat the procedure at the points on her back. She reports a slight "heavy," not unpleasant, feeling, mixed with relaxing drowsiness.

When the treatment is over, in slightly less than an hour, Rosemarie feels no unpleasant aftereffects. In fact she feels refreshed. This is the usual experience of my patients and is one of the reasons why they look forward to acupuncture visits without the usual dread reserved for conventional doctor visits. We then discuss a future series of treatments. Because hypertension is measured by taking blood pressure readings, I can record her reponse to each treatment. If her blood pressure goes down and stays down, she can be weaned off her medication gradually. By then, her other problems of difficulty sleeping, frequent urination, and stress will doubtless have been resolved.

After the first treatment, some patients may experience a small amount of symptomatic relief, no matter what their complaint. Other patients may improve dramatically. This "instant" improvement may be temporary, but subsequent treatments will give more prolonged improvement. In the average case, with continued treatment, the patient notices a steady disappearance of symptoms and a growing sense of well-being. Change usually takes place gradually, for most illnesses have developed over time. Each patient's rate of improvement is different, depending on age, the duration and seriousness of the condition, and the patient's general constitution.

This has been the case for Rosemarie. Over a four-month period with a weekly appointment, her blood pressure has fallen to within the normal range, and she no longer needs medication. She now has her pressure checked periodically and sees me six to eight times a year for a preventive program.

The effects of acupuncture visits can be "objectively" monitored or observed. Blood pressure reading, urine and blood sampling, and other tests can tell us if a problem is being reversed. For example, another patient of mine, Joe, contracted hepatitis B three years before seeing me. The problem had become chronic. The disease had changed, and his physician suspected that he now had severe liver damage. Joe's chief complaints were pain along the sides of his body, fatigue, and depression, and a daily, dull headache. His liver function readings had skyrocketed.

In the treatment plan we set up together, we worked out a new diet, herbal remedies to regenerate his liver, and weekly acupuncture sessions. Joe was a motivated patient. His internist had told him that there was virtually no cure for this form of hepatitis. He also learned that, if left unchecked, hepatitis could lead to cirrhosis, cancer, or liver failure. His doctor suggested he join an experimental program in which he would take a very expensive drug of questionable worth with many adverse side effects.

Joe tried acupuncture weekly for three months, and then every other week for five months. During this time, his liver function readings turned around. He was able to relax about the state of his health, and his pain and headaches subsided. As a bonus, he experienced relief from recurring herpes outbreaks. His last laboratory results showed all readings to be in the normal range. A year later he still maintains normal readings and feels "great."

What can acupuncture do for you that Western medicine cannot? A conventional doctor looks at a patient's body in terms of disease. He records sets of symptoms and orders appropriate tests and/or X-rays so that he can isolate specific causes. Once a cause has been established, he uses procedures, usually intrusive, to destroy or remove diseased tissue or to reconstruct a faulty body part. His focus is always narrow and specific. Western medicine is specialized and lacks an overview of the whole person.

To a doctor trained in Traditional Chinese Medicine, a patient is not a "hypertension case" or a "hepatitis case," but rather a whole person. The illness that brings a person to consultation is not something that just needs to be isolated and removed, but is a reflection of an underlying disharmony in the total body makeup. We in Traditional Chinese Medicine do not specialize: each of us is extensively and intensively trained in the same four-thousand-year-old body of knowledge and art of healing. When we gently touch one of your diagnostic points, noting carefully the gradation of its response, it is to collect a subtle clue as to the working of your body—perhaps in a place far distant from the actual place of touch. Taken together, these bits of evidence help determine a program of needle placement that will restore your body's natural harmony. Indeed, harmony and health are synonymous to the acupuncturist. Thus, although Western medicine sets strict limits on what is to be included in diagnosis, thereby excluding many symptoms, an acupuncture diagnosis includes information of almost unlimited scope.

Although acupuncture treatment is subtle, its effects continue to be felt long after the needles are removed. It can improve blood flow, change fluid distribution, generate electrical nerve impulses, and stimulate brain cells. Later in this book, I will describe how needles work: making glands secrete, decreasing or increasing body chemicals and ion pressure, and stimulating areas of the brain. In short, acupuncture builds a healing environment.

Like Western medicine, Traditional Chinese Medicine is a system of diagnosis and treatment. We practitioners of Traditional Chinese Medicine use Western diagnostic tools: blood tests, e-span or X-ray tests, and so on, but these techniques are never more than adjuncts to our work. Ultimately, we rely on the diagnostic methods developed over the centuries. Our treatment consists of acupuncture sessions over a period of time and the ongoing checking of symptoms, pulses, point sensitivities, and tongue changes.

NOTE

1. Ric Carlson, *The End of Medicine*, New York: Wiley, 1975, 70–71.

REFERENCES

For information on patient care, see M. Porkett and C. Ullman, *Chinese Medicine: Its History, Philosophy, and Practice and Why It May One Day Dominate the Medicine of the West* (1982). Also useful are *The Meridians of Acupuncture* (1981) by Felix Mann and *Acupuncture Case Histories From China* (1988), edited by Chen Jirui and Nissi Wang.

Chapter 3

HOW ACUPUNCTURE WORKS FROM A CHINESE VIEW

The ancient Chinese believed that the human body is a continuum of energy ranging between two poles. One pole is called *yin* and the other *yang*. Although yin and yang are at opposite ends of the continuum, they continually interact with one another. When a person is healthy, a harmonious balance is struck in the amount of energy exchanged between yin and yang; neither pole dominates the other. When a person is ill, excess energy has accumulated in the direction of one pole, thereby leaving the other pole deficient in its share. Disease and injury are considered states of imbalance between yin and yang. The job of medicine is to restore and sustain the delicate balance between the poles.

This balance can be thought of as homeostasis—the condition of any system that is self-correcting and self-regulating. The temperature falls below or rises above a comfortable level—one's "thermostat" turns the furnace on or off to restore an ideal temperature. The balance can be changed (within limits), but if the system fails, a repair person must be called in to fix it. Of course, the concept of homeostasis does appear in

Western medicine: Balances are sought in the endocrine system, between ions such as sodium and potassium, and in pH balance.

But a Traditional Chinese Medical doctor thinks of illness differently from the way most Western physicians conceive it. In the West, the doctor hopes to "cure" a problem after people are unbearably sick, when they are in pain or feel physically disruptive symptoms. A traditional Chinese practitioner, by contrast, seeks to prevent disease by keeping all systems balanced and finely tuned throughout the patient's life span. Consultation with the practitioner of acupuncture is ideally an ongoing part of every patient's life. Although the idea of preventive medicine (for instance, prenatal care) is prominent in current discussions about revamping our medical care system, there is really no comparison to the prevention that is accomplished through acupuncture and herbs.

We practitioners trained in Traditional Chinese Medicine know that extreme changes in the environment, such as prolonged exposure to heat or cold, can cause sudden illness. Illness also comes from a gradual blocking and deficiency of body energy. We see the body threatened by lifestyle factors such as overeating or overworking. We also look for disharmonies of the internal nature in intensely prolonged emotional states such as grief or depression.

Serious consequences follow when yin and yang remain imbalanced for excessive periods, beyond the body's natural capacity to (homeostatically) readjust. Excess yang and deficient yin—or vice versa—throw the normal body out of balance and cause illness. If this condition persists and progresses to the point where there is a total collapse of energies, death results. The role of acupuncture is to provide a correcting outside influence that will restore balance.

Although I spoke of yin and yang as poles, they are not literal locations in the body. Rather, they are dynamic states that continually create and regulate one another through many subtle transformations. You cannot inhale without exhaling—one actions passes into the others and back again. You cannot flex a muscle without soon relaxing it. If you overexert the muscles of your arm, you will feel a cramp in that arm (excess energy); the cramp will not go away until you temporarily stop using the arm, thereby drawing off the energy to restore the balance. Yin and yang define and constrain one another by striking a balance between excess and deficient energy levels. They are fluid states of beginning, acting, changing, resting—in short, the entire repertoire of balances that constitutes being.

Within these broad yin and yang categories, there are possibilities for fine-tuning balances. For example, at one level, cold weather is considered yin and hot is yang. Yet within cold, there are degrees and stages of cold: very cold is yin, and moderately cold, in comparison, is yang. Cold in the body is a yin illness that will appear to the sufferer as steady, localized pain; but within the yin there may be yang-like experiences of pain, manifested as very sharp, intermittent contractions. Heat in the body is yang illness, such as a bad case of influenza; an accompanying loss of weight and weakness are yin qualities of an essentially yang illness. In the Chinese view, there are balances within balances, and this complex dynamic is the province of the Traditional Medical practitioner.

To restore balance and harmony, the physician observes and measures how, where, when, and why the yin and yang got out of whack. Having established the nature of a disharmony, the physician then inserts needles into points on the surface of the body that directly affect what goes on deep inside it. Needling alters the activities of the many energies—the *Chi*—that travel through distinct pathways in the body called meridians.

The operation of all the body's systems hinge on Chi. Sickness is a deviation or misdirection of the Chi energy and not a separate happening. Chi is world pervasive: all "things," "seasons," systems," "states of being" —everything of this word is formed and kept whole and true by this energy. Chi energy is recognized by its acts and results. Our Chi comes to us at birth as part of our acquired essence. After birth, Chi is accumulated, enriched, and balanced by food and air. Thus, the original Chi is in the adult balanced with acquired Chi's. In illness, blocked Chi reacts in predictable ways and produces predictable results. So does Chi that is depleted or running wildly out of control.

Chi is also the Chinese name given to the sensation a patient feels in the area where the needle is inserted. There is no exact equivalent for the term in English, but it can be translated as "to take." "Taking" is what happens when one starts driving a nail into wood; at a precise moment, the nail bites into the surface. We could equally well say that the wood bites the nail; it separates its fibers and closes them around the nail, grasping it. The acupuncturist feels the Chi in her fingertips and a tightening around the needle. The Chi felt by the patients can be any one of a combination of delicate sensations: slight numbness, tingling, heaviness, faint and brief soreness, warmth, or a minute electrical shock. Patients who are accustomed to the acupuncturist's care can even assist in the practitioner's accurate placement of the needle. The patient may say, "I do (or don't yet) feel the Chi," or "the Chi is too strong now."

Over many centuries of trial and error, practitioners evolved a formal system of needle points. They discovered that points lined up into distinct pathways, which they called channels or meridians. These meridians took recognized courses, not only along the surface of the body, but also within it at many levels, through tissue and muscles, into the organs themselves.

Meridian is the English translation of a French translation of the Chinese term meaning "pathway." Meridians are analogous to the threads that make up a fabric, interconnecting and forming it into a network. We speak of meridians as an invisible network that links all parts of the body together, the pathways over which energy travels. The theory of points and meridians lies at the very foundation of acupuncture medicine.

It took about sixteen hundred years, between 200 and 1800 a.d., before all of the acupuncture points were discovered and named. We now know their locations on the body, as well as the depths at which we need to insert the needles to reach the Chi. Knowledge is still accumulating about the specific effects each point yields. Extra, off-pathway points are still being discovered. Meridian routes are standardized in twelve main meridians, fifteen collaterals, and eight extraordinary channels.

Meridians integrate all the body's energies by connecting with one another and by relating various organs and organ functions. For example, the Lung meridian has direct and indirect effects on the lungs, but it also influences respiration, general energy level, coughs of all kinds, nasal passages, normal and abnormal perspiration, and some aspects of elimination. We use the Lung meridian to treat lung problems directly, but we also use it in conjunction with Kidney meridians for certain kinds of asthma and coughs. In addition to the Large Intestine meridian, the Lung meridian helps to treat skin ailments. Problems arising along the actual meridian path come under its domain: temperature changes felt along the meridian surface, increased/decreased sensitivity in areas or points, swellings and discolorations on the skin, and other changes. Such conditions are road signs that dictate the direction of an acupuncturist's treatment and locations of the needle insertions. In this way, the practitioner organizes signs (what the doctor observes) and symptoms (what the patent feels) into an overall diagnosis.

Let me describe the workings of a single representative acupuncture point called Spleen 6. This major point is located at a precisely measured distance above the ankle bone (on the inside edge), and at the back of the tibia, the larger of the two long bones of the lower leg. The Chinese name, *San Yin Chiao*, specifies the point's very essence: it is at the junction of the three yin meridians on the leg: the Spleen, Liver, and Kidney meridians. Spleen 6 is crucial in women's diseases: here one treats all kinds of menstrual disorders. It can also be used to correct abnormal fetal position and to induce labor. Spleen 6 plays a part in certain male disorders as well, including premature ejaculation and involuntary emission of semen. For both sexes, the Spleen 6 point can be needled to alleviate hypertension, migraine headaches, kidney inflammation, paralysis of the leg, bleeding, hemorrhoids, weakness in the stomach, and painful urination, to list a few. Modern medical research shows that stimulating Spleen 6 activates the autonomic reflex circuit. This means that needling the Spleen 6 point can cause nerves to conduct impulses from the peripheral areas (limbs) toward the central nervous system. It can also stimulate impulses from the brain or spinal cord to the peripheral system, such as the leg. Spleen 6 has been shown to stimulate the cells that secrete insulin, and it decreases sugar in the blood.

Disturbances along the Spleen meridian itself—indicating imbalances—can cause symptoms such as nausea, vomiting, pain along the pathway, and abdominal distention (along with belching and/or flatulence). The patient feels weak, heavy, and sluggish and may have decreased appetite and diarrhea. The practitioner may see signs along the meridian such as discolorations, tenderness to touch, or pitting (marked with a shallow depression under pressure).

Spleen 6 influences certain body functions and energy balances because of the pathway its meridian takes. It travels from the great toe along the inside edge of the foot, up the inner side of the leg and thigh, through the inguinal area and abdomen until it reaches the spleen itself. It has branches inside the body that connect it to the stomach, heart, upper chest, neck, larynx, the back of the tongue, and the glands of the mouth. Therefore, acupuncturists use the point for treating leg edema, fibroid tumors and cysts in the uterus or abdominal cavity, cardiac edema, and abdominal pain.

The meridians or channels are not the only energy system; the organ systems that receive, rejuvenate, rebuild, and recalculate the energies are another. These organ systems have names in Traditional Chinese medicine similar to those in Western practice: Kidney, Liver, Heart, Spleen, and Lung. The systems are actually domains that have very broad powers and influences not only on the particular organ they are associated with but also on the overall physiological aspects of the organ. Each system has effects in the entire body.

Looking at the Kidney system, we see that its energy is responsible for the development, integrity, and daily workings of the central nervous system, the brain, and the muscular-skeletal, reproductive, and urinary systems. It controls all of the developmental stages of life from birth to death. In addition, it underlies or supports all the other systems, and in conjunction with the Heart, Lungs, Liver, and Spleen, it keeps us alive. It is the source of all genetic material, and ultimately it influences all cellular life. In the Traditional Chinese view, it is the deep and slow-moving water energy, the most essential of all body processes.

Kidney energies, in collaboration with other systems, regulate the body's innumerable metabolic processes. Chinese physicians saw a correspondence between Kidney and Heart energy long before Western medicine discovered the role of these two organs in regulating blood pressure.

They also recognized an intimate Kidney-Lung relationship—a nurturing mist of energy that keeps the lungs strong and clear. For example, Traditional Chinese Medicine often sees childhood asthma as a manifestation of early Kidney malfunctioning, spilling over into the Lung's domain.

The Kidney and Liver relationship is one of the body's most intimate. The closeness between the two systems can be recognized in their functions: The Kidney system generates energy, and the Liver system circulates it. If you think of the Liver system as the powerhouse and the Kidney system as the pumping system, you can grasp the importance of each to every other critical system and subsystem.

One of the main functions of the Liver energy system is storage of Blood. (I use a capital letter to designate organ systems in their broadest, most inclusive sense.) The Liver system controls nourishment through this Blood, and it regulates actions such as the building, breakdown, cleaning, and recycling of tissue. In Traditional Chinese Medicinal theory, it is the foremost line of defense against stress, whether physical, chemical, or emotional. Because of its close relationship to Blood, the Liver system has the capacity to restore itself and, therefore, the body as a whole. It is, so to speak, a mediator between signal and response. Here's how it works. An emotion triggers the nervous system, alerting the Kidney system through the thyroid and adrenal glands (the endocrine system is a function of Kidney and Spleen energy), which sends signals to the Liver system. The Liver system circulates a flow of energy that activates the spleen system, moving energy to the mind (the Spleen's domain), as well as activating the Blood to move muscles and nerves into physical action. Thus, the Blood system nourishes and oversees the working of the body's muscles and nerves. Receiving, interpreting, and reacting to any stimulation is a complex and integrated process that is dependent on the Liver channel. A patient labeled as "stuck" in Traditional Chinese Medicine has a Liver channel imbalance, preventing him from making decisions.

The Heart channel and its energies embody the soul or Spirit of the person. Through these energies, we "grow" in awareness and mental ability. These energies influence all the highest aspects of life: creativity, love, and divine inspiration. The Heart channel controls the circulation of these ideas around the body through its intimate connections with the two trunk channels, known as the Pericardium and the Triple Warmer.

The inhibition of Heart energy by shock or some great emotional trauma will, in turn, affect the Spirit and the circulation. Early practitioners recognized the Heart's role in maintaining the nervous system, circulation, sleep, mental health, and creativity.

Next, the Spleen system dedicates itself to the survival of the individual through digestion, absorption, and metabolic breakdown of real substances like food and water. (Note that the Spleen system is different from the Spleen 6, which is a point on a meridian.) It transforms food and water into necessary energy. A body that cannot metabolize food efficiently cannot thrive. The Spleen energy feeds all the other organs. It is also the seat of what Westerners call the ego, and it begins its work in utero along with the Kidney. Dysfunctions in either system can lead to many developmental defects. Postpartum shock to the Spleen can induce physical problems throughout life. These problems appear in digestive and elimination systems. In the brain, these shocks can cause difficulty in assimilating information. Incoherence, illogical thinking, fixed ideas, lack of concentration, and the inability to communicate are all the later mental stages of poorly developed Spleen energy. The Western idea that malnutrition can cause poor mental development was known to Chinese Medicine millennia ago.

Finally, there is the organ system called Lung. From our first breath, Lung energy ensures our existence on this earth. The Lung nourishes and strengthens our physical being. Dysfunction of energy in the chest interferes with deep breathing and results in poor oxygenation of the blood. The patient experiencing this energy dysfunction complains of low energy.

Dr. Leon Hammer sees the energy system of all these organ

channels as an integrated, functioning whole. He speaks of a flowering of self: self-esteem, self-confidence, independence, responsibility, strength, and the ability to learn from failure. He says that the Kidney provides courage to face the unknown, the Liver gives direction, the Heart allows expression of self, the Spleen encourages compassion, and the Lung gives impetus for moving to new levels of self. Thus, Traditional Chinese Medicine takes into acount the complete person—physically, mentally, and spiritually. When I practice this medicine, I see my patients in their entirety. I can take many pieces of information, often seemingly unrelated, and piece them together to form a coherent diagnosis. Grasping the nature of underlying chaos, I can turn the tide of the disease.

Thousands of years ago, needles were made of ordinary stone. Later, they were made of more precious materials, such as jade. Common metals like iron were used, as were gold and silver. Needles were even make of bamboo. In recent archaeological excavations in China, scientists found nine different kinds of acupuncture needles, along with heavier three-sided prismatic needles used for drawing blood. The dating of the needles places their use as early as 1000 b.c.

Modern acupuncture needles are made of stainless surgical steel and are very thin and flexible. They vary in length from one-half to five inches and in thickness from 25 to 32 gauge. Short needles are likely to be used on areas such as the face, head, hands, and feet. Medium-length needles are used on the abdomen, chest, back, and limbs. On very fleshy areas of the body like the buttocks, longer needles can be used. The needles have a dowel end, rather than a cutting tip like that of a hypodermic needle. They rarely cause tissue damage, bleeding or bruising. The acupuncturist, as noted earlier, inserts the needle quickly, using a steady hand movement, or else aims it through a tiny tube.

We acupuncturists take great pride in our insertion technique. We practice on objects like rubber balls and fruit, or on ourselves and our fellow students, to develop wrist, hand, and finger strength. We also perfect coordination between eye and hand, fingers and tool. Every student must master rigorous standards for fast, painless, and accurate needle insertion. It is an intensive part of our training.

There is absolutely no danger that a patient may contract any diseases that might be transmitted by nonsterile or inadequately cleaned needles. Once acupuncturists began to grind, polish, and sterilize their own needles, they developed a fondness for them akin to what musicians feel for their instruments or what cabinetmakers feel for their fine tools.

Until recently, they maintained their own needles, even making them from scratch, and swapping information about needles was part of every acupuncturist's professional life. Today needles are standardized, and most of them are disposable.

Acupuncture is far from being a static medical practice. Many new and exciting discoveries are constantly being tested.

Drug needling is another Western/Eastern marriage. It involves injecting a small dose of an herbal medicine or a vitamin into acupuncture points. A much smaller quantity of medicine is used than if taken orally or given by hypodermic injection. For example, in cases of neurological disorders, B vitamin is the usual vitamin injection. In gynecological cases, angelica (the Chinese herb Tang Kuei) is injected into an acupuncture point.

Magnetic therapy refers both to the application of magnets directly to points and to magnetic-electric acupuncture, which is done with wires connecting points to magnets. Sometimes magnets are left on the points, and the patient "wears" them, so that stimulation continues uninterruptedly after the patient leaves the practitioner's office. I have used these magnets to treat pain. Some practitioners use magnets on cancer cases, over areas of tumor sites, or on points stimulating immune-enhancing activity.

In magnetic-electric acupuncture, needles are replaced by magnets connected to a simple machine that supplies a small amount of electric current. The effects are similar to those of needling, and the technique can be especially helpful when treating children or hypersensitive adults. Although some very interesting and promising results have been reported with magnetic therapy, it is a new treatment and is not yet a routine part of most acupuncturists' practice.

Laser acupuncture replaces the needle with a light beam. A laser ray is intense, extremely narrow, and can be aimed with extraordinary precision. Low intensity and cold light make up an acupuncture laser. There is no burning or destruction of tissue. In Germany, laser acupuncture is now being used satisfactorily to treat chronic leg ulcers, wounds that resist healing, herpes zoster scars, neuralgias, and stomach inflammations. The laser is quite safe, reduces treatment time by 90 percent, and is completely painless. I have used laser acupuncture on babies, very young children, and small pets with great success. It causes no trauma or tears. Laser acupuncture does have one disadvantage: the required equipment is expensive and difficult to have serviced in this country.

Laser acupuncture is effective in treating skin and scalp problems. Some of my fellow practitioners have had very good success in treating alopecia areata (loss of head hair in sharply defined patches). I treated one case of alopecia areata that responded well to a dozen treatment sessions.

Traditional Chinese Medicine utilizes a highly developed body of knowledge about medicinal herbs. These herbs may be applied externally in the form of salves, or as drops and powders to be dissolved in liquids and drunk. Herbs can be cooked into a medicinal soup or dried, ground, and put into a gelatin capsule. These herbal medicines should only be prescribed by a practitioner who has been schooled in their use. They are true medicines and have a pharmacology all their own. Each herb has unique properties, side effects, and correct therapeutic values. One special herb—artemisia—is burned directly or indirectly on the acupuncture points. No pain is felt during this procedure, which is called "moxibustion."

This mugwort (in Latin, *Artemisia Vulgaris*) is the principal herb used in acupuncture and has a distinct odor when lit. It is sometimes used in combination with other herbs to make a "God's Needle," a cigar-shaped stub that can be ignited.

This stub glows, much like incense does when lit. Acupuncturists hold the glowing tip against the head of the needle in order to conduct heat into the point. When used indirectly, we pinch a very small amount of mugwort into a cone, place it on the skin, and ignite it. The herb (also called moxa) is allowed to glow just until the patient starts to feel warmth; then it is quickly removed so as not to burn the skin. Moxa heat has been discovered to be especially effective in relieving certain types of pain, such as that associated with sprains, bursitis, tendonitis, and arthritis.

The technique of moxibustion—the burning of mugwort moxa—is as old as acupuncture itself. It is still used because it works. Traditional Chinese Medicine shares with Western science a strong empirical bent; if a medication or procedure has positive results and no negative side effects, it will be used in treatment, even though the underlying reasons for its success may not be fully understood.

REFERENCES

Specific channel information can be found in the series *Chinese Medicine from the Classic: The Lung; the Kidney; the Spleen, etc.* by C. Larre and E. R. de La Vallee, in Felix Mann's book *Acupuncture: The Ancient*

Chinese Art of Healing and How It Works Scientifically (1973), *Acupuncture: A Comprehensive Text* (1981), translated and edited by J. O'Conner and D. Bensky, and in the compilation by the Shanghai College of Traditional Medicine, *Essentials of Chinese Acupuncture*. Dr. James Tin Yao So's *The Book of Acupuncture Points* (1984) is also informative.

For additional reading in traditional Chinese Medicine theory, see G. Maciocia, *The Foundations of Chinese Medicine* (1989), or the book by L. Hammer, M.D., *Dragon Rises—Red Bird Flies* (1990). *Modern Chinese Acupuncture* (1983) by G. T. Lewith and N. R. Lewith is very comprehensive.

For herbal medicine theory and practice, a good place to start is *Chinese Herbal Medicine*, compiled and translated by Bensky and Gable (1986). Low's and Turner's 1981 book *The Principle and Practice of Moxibustion* (1981) offers a good, though specialized, treatment of the subject.

Chapter 4

HOW ACUPUNCTURE
WORKS FROM A WESTERN VIEW

Chinese explanations of how acupuncture works are rooted in Chinese medical philosophy and theory. Eastern concepts about causality do not have specific counterparts in Western science. Thus, terms like yin/yang and Chi do not have exact English equivalents. "No-nonsense" Western scientists are uncomfortable with concepts like the "harmonious balance of energies" that the Eastern theorists and practitioners use to describe a healthy body.

Our scientists want to get at what is "really" going on when an acupuncture treatment gets results. They want to describe the process in the scientific jargon with which they are familiar. Westerners believe they can "see" how a process operates when it can be broken down into elements that can be named and measured in the laboratory: electrical current, chemical compounds, and substances whose size, shape, and temperature can be described.

There is a certain arrogance in this approach. We (in the West) it seems will tell them (the Chinese) what they are doing, since they are themselves ignorant of the scientific basis for their activity. Their (Chinese) explanations and theories are mystifications. We sometimes forget that in our own medicine we have often accepted cures that have eluded explanation for generations.

Our use of analgesics is a good example. For at least twenty-five hundred years, the opium poppy was cultivated and used to induce sleep and to soothe pain. In 1806 morphine was discovered to be the active ingredient in opium, and soon Western physicians began to use it to treat pain. We have eagerly welcomed other painkillers like aspirin, which was extracted from tree bark at least as far back as ancient Roman times. Yet, even though opium and aspirin have been used for generations to ease pain, scientists did not begin to understand how either worked in the human body until about twenty-five years ago. Neither physicians nor patients cared whether or not the physiological mechanism through which these drugs killed pain was known. That they eased pain was certain, and this was enough for anyone who suffered.

To understand in Western scientific terms how acupuncture and herbal medicine works is a prodigious undertaking. In this chapter, I will consider the causes and treatment of pain because this aspect of acupuncture has received the most attention in the West. More study is needed in other areas of biochemistry, for example, in endocrinology, to get a complete picture of how needling affects the various body systems. For the moment, we have evidence of how and why acupuncture works to relieve pain. In a later chapter, I will describe how pain is being treated, both in my practice and in clinics around the world.

For three thousand years, acupuncture has been used to treat pain. Less than forty years ago, with the revival of Traditional Chinese Medicine in China, acupuncture was brought into modern operating rooms to control pain, during and after surgery. Western physicians learned of acupuncture's dramatic effectiveness when James Reston, journalist for the *New York Times*, wrote about his firsthand experience. Reston had gone to Beijing at the invitation of the Chinese government. During his visit, he had to undergo an emergency appendectomy. His Chinese doctors used acupuncture for his postoperative pain, and Reston recovered quickly. Upon his return to the United States, he wrote about his experience. As China opened its doors wider, delegations of Western doctors went to observe for themselves the "miracle" that traditional practitioners had been working there since 1000 B.C.

Just a few years later, in 1976, the actual mechanism by which morphine and aspirin kill pain was discovered. Scientists isolated a group of substances called endorphins that are released by the pituitary gland in the front part of the brain. Sites in the brain called receptors respond to these endorphins by blocking pain sensations. Substances such as aspirin and morphine and processes such as acupuncture stimulate the natural production of endorphins.

Our bodies manufacture endorphins under various conditions—for example, when we experience severe physical trauma or intense emotional stress. Injured motorists who climb out of their cars after a head-on collision often report that they were only aware of having to do something immediately. They say that they felt no pain until after the danger was past. In such instances, the body produces endorphins, numbing the pain until people can act to save themselves and get medical attention—which usually includes receiving "something for the pain."

Endorphins are chemical messengers of a type known as neuro-transmitters: They communicate between nerve cells. These cells (called neurons) are not connected physically to one another. Each neuron consists of a cell body, with a nucleus at the center, dendrites (very fine projections of cell body), and an axon (or the main projection along which impulses travel). Nerve impulses are electrical charges that travel from one end of the elongated neuron to the other, coming to a complete stop at the end of the axon. At the end of the axon is a gap called a synapse. Nerve impulses cannot jump across the synapse to the next nerve cell without the help of chemical transmitters—messengers that move the impulse across the gap. Neurotransmitters move at very high speeds and interact with specific receptors at the next nerve cell, passing information to them. Back and forth, again and again, the chemical messengers travel between the endings of adjacent neurons, transmitting impulses throughout the entire nervous system.

After the breakthrough discovery of endorphins in 1976, Dr. Bruce Pomeranz, a Canadian physician with a Ph.D. in neurobiology, conducted a series of experiments that provided the first evidence that acupuncture stimulates endorphin release. Dr. Pomeranz's work demonstrated that acupuncture analgesia was mediated through endorphins.

Pomeranz's early experiments dealt with drug addiction and the effects of withdrawal. He hypothesized that when morphine is injected into the body, the pituitary gland stops producing endorphins. That would explain why, when morphine is withdrawn from the system, the subject feels severe discomfort. The pituitary will not restart and begin producing its own endorphins until the level of morphine in the body is reduced to a level that allows the gland to function normally.

Pomeranz hypothesized that acupuncture killed pain by stimulating the release of endorphins. He performed a series of now classic experiments in which he needled rabbits. He discovered that their thresholds of pain rose when needled. Next, he circulated blood from these rabbits to other rabbits that had not been needled. Their pain thresholds also rose. He then removed the pituitary glands from a select group of rabbits to see if acupuncture analgesia could still be induced. As he suspected, no acupuncture analgesia could be induced in animals without glands.

Certain drugs (called morphine antagonists) can suppress the painkilling effects of morphine in the body. In subsequent experiments, Pomeranz administered one of these antagonists—naloxone—into the bodies of healthy rabbits. He then applied a powerful stimulus whose effects acupuncture could usually eliminate. But needling did not stop the pain. He concluded that because naloxone rendered both morphine and acupuncture ineffective as analgesics, it must have prevented the same normal action: that is, it must have blocked both the morphine and the acupuncture from releasing endorphins.

The next series of experiments was directed at measuring pain intensity and how well acupuncture could control it. Pomeranz and his co-workers observed that after needling, pain diminished somewhat after ten minutes, became minimal after about twenty minutes, and between twenty and sixty minutes after acupuncture no pain was felt at all. The different lengths of time required to bring about the pain-sedating effects are due to the existence of endorphins with different molecular forms. There are three kinds of endorphins: alpha-, beta-, and gamma-endorphins. The pain-relieving effects of alpha- and beta-endorphins are short-lived, peaking at about twenty minutes. The gamma-endorphins, however, may not reach their peak effectiveness for as long as four hours.

These differences account for the prolonged analgesic effects of acupuncture observed clinically and in surgical and postoperative situations. When acupuncture anesthesia is used for surgery, the alpha- and beta-endorphins require twenty to thirty minutes for analgesia to take effect. Gamma-endorphins are probably at work when the pain relief lasts after the operation is over.

When acupuncture is used in tooth extractions, patients rarely feel pain during, immediately following, or after the extraction. In over six thousand tooth extractions done at the Institute of Acupuncture at Colombo

South General Hospital, Sri Lanka, not a single case of postextraction pain was reported. Further, in more than twenty-five hundred major surgical procedures of many kinds carried out at the same hospital, patients who had received acupuncture required one-third less drugs postoperatively than those who received standard Western anesthesia.[1]

Recently, it has become possible to synthetically manufacture endorphins for use as drugs, but these endorphins are extremely unstable and are destroyed in the body in a matter of seconds. Moreover, synthetic endorphins cost about $30,000 per gram to manufacture. Acupuncture is considerably cheaper!

Chinese scientists are convinced that endorphin release is central to acupuncture analgesia because they have measured elevations of endorphins through radio wave analysis of the entire brain. But they are not convinced that endorphin release is the only mechanism involved. In recent years, additional neurotransmitters have been added to the list of natural substances whose release is stimulated by acupuncture therapy. These include serotonin, dopamine, epinephrine, norepinephrine, acetylcholine, glycine, gamma-aminobutyrill (GABA), and glutamate.

The belief that other neurotransmitters may be involved in needling effects is supported by evidence concerning some significant differences between morphine and acupuncture use. Morphine and other opiates depress respiratory functions; acupuncture does not. Acupuncture relieves constipation, bronchospasms, and gastrointestinal spasms; opiates have the opposite effect. Constriction of the eye's pupil is a characteristic effect of morphine-like substances; no such constriction occurs during acupuncture. Needling promotes the release of corticosteroid from the adrenal cortex; opiates depress the cortex.

Dr. Yoshiaki Omura of Manhattan College in New York City thinks that acupuncture may release a large molecule from the pituitary called adrenocorticotropic hormone (ACTH). The level of this substance stimulated by acupuncture may explain the prolonged pain relief provided for joint and motor disorders, both acute and chronic. Furthermore, increased serum serotonin levels may account for the relaxed, sleepy sensation that often follows acupuncture treatment.

Incidentally, researchers have discovered that certain strains of mice do not seem to respond to acupuncture; they genetically lack the necessary opiate receptors. Some people who do not respond to needling—a 10 percent minority—may fail to do so because they, too, genetically lack these requisite neural receptors.

These studies on the relationship between acupuncture and endorphins, neurochemicals, and opiate receptors suggest that needling works to treat problems other than pain.

A study of epilepsy, including traumatic epilepsy, suggests many mechanisms at work. Ninety-eight epileptics were treated by needling specific sedative acupuncture points. All drugs were discontinued during the first weeks of therapy, and treatments lasted from one to eighteen months. The subjects were 2 to 52 years old. Sixty-five cases showed marked improvement with an absence of epileptic attacks during a one-year period without drugs. Patients received maintenance treatments of acupuncture once every two or three months after a cure was effected. Follow-up was either by letter or visits for the next six years. Relapses occurred in only five cases.[2]

Acupuncture has been useful in treating skin wounds and in promoting the healing of scars. It also lowers concentrations of potassium ion, histamine, and bradykinin in the peripheral blood. Again, research shows that aspirin and certain amino acids enhance the action of acupuncture, suggesting that other neurochemicals could be involved in the effect.

The role of acupuncture in pain management is being reexamined in the light of new knowledge about the nervous system. The time lag between needling and various stages of pain relief suggests that a neurotransmitter mechanism such as endorphin release is a better explanation than any other current hypothesis. One theory suggests that the large, myelinated nerve fibers in the central nervous system that convey information about touch, pressure, and deep sensations use one kind of transmitter to do so, while the thin unmyelinated nerve fibers in the same system may be using another kind of transmitter. Acupuncture-stimulated sensations travel through both the large and small fibers. Both nerve fiber sets end in the central nervous system at the spinal cord, in an area rich in opiate receptors.

Another hypothesis suggests that the autonomic nervous system (ANS) plays a role in acupuncture. The ANS controls impulses to those parts of the body we do not consciously control, such as the heart, glands, and digestion. Evidence shows that some acupuncture impulses do, in fact, travel to the spinal cord and to the brain along blood vessels that are part of the ANS. Research on this phenomenon is ongoing.

Only one theory so far proposed encompasses many of the diverse effects that acupuncture produces: the thalamic neuron theory of Yang Feng and Ren Shizen at the Zhongguo Medical College in China. This theory comprises an intriguing set of hypotheses that explain a broad range of clinical observations on needling. Proposed in 1978, the theory states that if any peripheral pathology occurs in the body, there is a corresponding abnormal activity in the brain. When acupuncture stimulates the targeted cells in the brain through needling points peripheral to the brain, it normalizes the activity of these cells. This normalization is accomplished by repeated stimulation not unlike the phenomenon of psychological conditioning.

Another proposed theory suggests that ancient acupuncture channels are closely related to the distribution network of the peripheral nerves. Starting at the embryonic stage, nerve supply patterns continually differentiate and shift, arranging and rearranging themselves from primitive to more complex nerve bundles. Every embryo begins with forty-two pairs of "somites" or cell masses. These somites contain three components: a *somatic* part that will develop into limbs and trunk, muscle and bone; a *splanchnic* part that will differentiate into different body organs; and a *spinal* component that will unite all three parts into a functional whole. But no matter how complex these relationships and plexi become, each regional area supplied by the nerve segment will remain unchanged, retaining some of the cells it had in common with past embryonic cell mates. A fully developed human contains many specialized organs and tissue structures, all of which communicate with one another. Anatomists find that energy meridians and the majority of acupuncture points coincide with the spinal segments that connect these three parts. The pattern surely cannot be accidental.

Acupuncture has demonstrated its effectiveness in relieving many kinds of pain—from burning skin pain, to deep organ pain, to the stabbing pain of migraine. All of these kinds and locations of pain obviously do not operate by the same mechanisms, nor are their sensations connected to the central nervous system by identical peripheral nerve fibers. Nor do the nerve fibers traveled terminate in the same paths along the spinal cord. Yet acupuncture addresses all these types of pain. Through the hundreds of needle points, every cell in every type of tissue in the body can be reached.

No completely satisfactory explanation of the effectiveness of needling yet exists. All researchers in the field stress the urgent need for continued research in many directions. Some scientists are examining acupuncture in relation to the cardiovascular system; others are exploring the immunological or microcirculation systems for clues. No explanation has yet been found for some of the spectacular successes of acupuncture—

the recovery from paralysis and the cure of psoriasis, for example. A multifaceted, multidisciplinary approach is needed to unravel the mysteries of acupuncture.

The study of pain has provided only one avenue to understanding the general phenomenon of acupuncture. Researchers are investigating how various parts of the body are connected, how they communicate, and how distress in one area affects other areas. Further research is needed in body chemistry, the electrical functioning of the nerve cells, and the nervous system as a whole. With acupuncture, we must conceive of the body as a system of complex interdependencies, which is precisely the viewpoint that Traditional Chinese Medicine has emphasized for thousands of years.

Aspirin, morphine, and acupuncture all seem to work in similar ways to inhibit pain. This is stunning news, for if the human body responds similarly to apparently different treatments, then there are alternative treatments for pain. Acupuncture should therefore be considered a genuine medical alternative to use of these drugs. In many ways, it is the superior choice because acupuncture does not have the side effects that drugs have.

NOTES

1.   Anton Jayasuriya. "A Scientific Review of Acupuncture." *Seventh World Congress*, Oct. 1981. Meeting paper.
2.   Si Ziyu, et al. "The Efficacy of Electro-Acupuncture on 98 Cases of Epilepsy." *Chinese Acupuncture and Moxibustion.* 6 (1):17-18, 1986.

REFERENCES

Dr. Pomeranz's work and other scientific research into acupuncture is compiled in Pomeranz and Stux, *Scientific Bases of Acupuncture* (1988).

Part 2

ACUPUNCTURE AT WORK

Chapter 5

RELEASE FROM PAIN

We all suffer from physical pain at some time in our lives. Most of these episodes disappear with time, and with recuperation comes normalcy. For some, however, the episode takes on major consequences.

Tom suffered a work accident when a gas tank fell on his back. He underwent surgery twice for his injury, but that was not the end of it; he had several more procedures to block the nerves that kept him in constant, excruciating pain. Thoroughly disabled, Tom could not work or lead a normal daily existence. He was in costly rehabilitation hospitals under the care of physical therapists, psychologists, and nurses who trained him in the use of pain management; he was expected to learn to live with pain. He took several series of narcotic drugs with lengthy adjustments and readjustments of dosages in a futile attempt to find one that worked. He was an inpatient at several well-known pain clinics. Finally, these various cures themselves became a problem requiring treatment; he entered a detoxification center to withdraw from the painkillers to which he had become addicted.

The trail to recovery was interminable, first from the injury itself and then from its pain, and there was no end in sight. At this stage in the ordeal (three years after the original injury) and against the advice of his doctors, Tom came to see me. His chief complaint was low back pain at the site of the trauma and the surgery, as well as pain in his right leg. He described the leg pain as electric shocks running up and down his leg ceaselessly. He begged me to try to help him control the leg problem, which kept him from sleeping. I inserted needles at several points between the right hip and foot. Tom lay still on my table for twenty minutes while the needles unobtrusively did their work. When I removed them, the pain was gone. His leg never bothered him again,

Tom's experience is not unique. I have often been asked to treat pain that has not responded to conventional medical treatment.

Vic, a construction worker, was a similar case. He had surgery for a neck injury caused by a falling chunk of building material. The operation left him with pain on the left side of his head and face—pain that persisted for fifteen long years. Pain was his daily companion, starting from the moment he arose in the morning and increasing through the day. He had lost his appetite and suffered sleepless nights. He said that he had even banged his head against the wall for relief. When I first saw him in my office he was holding his face, digging his fingers into his forehead, scalp, eye, and cheek. We began a series of twenty treatments that lasted for five weeks. At their conclusion, Vic was his former self, free from pain. He visited my office, smiling and jaunty. He was enjoying the simple pleasure of uninterrupted sleep for the first time in years. His confidence and self-assurance returned, and he began looking for work.

Not all chronic pain conditions arise from accidents. Sometimes, simple and accustomed daily activities can produce them. Dr. Edgar Berman, in his book *The Solid Gold Stethoscope*, wryly observes that "one low back problem beginning from a number 2 iron swing on the water hole on a damp autumn morning can last a lifetime and cost a fortune."[1] Puttering around the garden, cleaning house, or mild recreational activity can all produce painful conditions that stubbornly resist every effort to correct them. Eighty percent of us will experience back pain, one of the most common forms of persistent discomfort. On any given day in the United States, six and half million people will be in bed nursing back pain. Only 10 percent of these six and half million aching backs have structural conditions that require surgery. The remainder are enduring pain due to excessive strain, years of poor body mechanics, and minor injuries—in short, the wear and tear of everyday life.

One obstacle to treating pain—which is a subjective experience—

is, of course, that it can't be observed by medical practitioners in the way injury or disease can be seen and examined. Patients can only report their experience, and doctors must trust that the pain is real and not just in "in the head" of the sufferer. Insofar as pain is a symptom of some other condition, an alarm that signals a treatable pathology, it serves a useful purpose. But when pain can't be traced to an identifiable organic cause, it becomes a problem in itself. This is the chronic version of pain that is so intractable. Elaborate and costly pain treatment centers attack the problem in numerous ways, employing the expertise of many branches of medicine and psychology. The treatment they offer is expensive, prolonged, and, sadly, often ineffective. It is impossible to measure pain, and therefore impossible also to define when it has been "cured." What they strive for is to restore some of the patient's functioning—to get him or her back to work or to social living in spite of pain. The goal is to teach the person to endure and tolerate pain, not to achieve freedom from it.

No wonder acupuncture has enjoyed growing acceptance as an alternative solution to pain reduction. In fact, of the many ills, injuries, and pathologies that acupuncture is used to treat, it has been employed for pain relief the most. Its reputation has spread in the United States through a grassroots consumer movement—by word of mouth—rather than by physicians' recommendations and referrals.

Earlier, I discussed how Western Chinese scientists explain how acupuncture relieves pain. Modern experimental research has confirmed and rationalized in Western terms what Eastern medicine has known for centuries. Some researchers and practitioners compare needling to repairing a computer system. When circuits malfunction, the first corrective measure is to send a burst through the system to clear the circuits of unwanted reverberating patterns. The inserted needles send energy messages through the nervous system, clearing the body of overloaded signals.

Each successive treatment continues to stimulate endorphin and enkephalin processes that provide both short- and long-term relief from pain. What is more, the needling stimulates anti-inflammatory agents similar to steroids that act directly on damaged nerves. Acupuncture has still other beneficial long-term effects, including eliminating excess fluids, increasing circulation in pain areas, and cleansing out the debris of dead cells and tissue. Thus, there is a bonus to acupuncture: there is not only release from pain but also healing of the underlying condition. Western-trained doctors who have even the slightest familiarity with acupuncture cannot and do not deny its effectiveness in alleviating pain. In my practice I am frequently called on to help people with long-standing and urgent torment. A few examples from my case files provide an idea of the wide variety in the types and locations of pain I have treated with acupuncture.

Betty received a whiplash injury in a car accident. Two years later, she was still having shooting pain in her neck, and there was referred pain running down her back, passing through her left shoulder and up through her face. For the neck, shoulder, and face, I needled the appropriate points. For her back, I performed a special type of Chinese massage and applied heat to the area. After three treatments, all of her symptoms disappeared.

Angela is a professional dancer who hurt her back during a performance. The back eventually healed itself, as happens with people who are physically fit, but Angela was left with pain in the upper thighs and buttocks that would not go away. Five treatments were sufficient to remove the persistent pain, although after dance practices she still experienced stiffness and twinges of discomfort. We continued needle treatments for a few more visits, and she now dances pain free.

Bill could barely manage the few stairs to my office for his first appointment. He was in obvious pain and wore house slippers because he could not bend to tie his shoelaces. He sat down awkwardly and told of years of pain. Hard physical labor was not required of him, but his work as a college professor was impaired. He had seen a parade of doctors, physical therapists, and a chiropractor. He listed all the drugs he had been given to ease his pain. He told me that the pain had become so bad that he sometimes passed out at his desk. And then he started to cry. He had come to the limits of his endurance and despaired of ever living a normal life again.

With the first visit, I began a program of needling, and Bill began to improve. The change was not instantaneous—his case was far too advanced to expect that—but gradually and steadily over the next three weeks he started having unaccustomed pain-free days. After two months of sessions he was joyfully living like the old Bill. He rode his bicycle to classes, put in long hours with his students, and even gave an end-of-the term party. He had more to celebrate than just the end of another school year.

Lucille came to me at the age of 32, having suffered wracking migraine headaches since she was a teenager. Over the years, the pattern of the attacks fluctuated from one each week to intervals of one every few months. With an air of defeat, she said, "I am weary of being out of the picture, not being able to work or take care of my children and my house. My life revolves around the headaches. When they come, they build up to violent throbbing on the side of my head. My eyes get so sensitive I can't stand light. I look sick. I feel sick. I just want to get into bed and sleep." The story Lucille tells of her ordeal is a familiar one, and so is the outcome.

With an acupuncture treatment program of twelve visits lasting eight weeks, she became headache free. Every two to three months, she returns for follow-up treatment to maintain her equilibrium and ensure her life of freedom from pain.

Margaret was a graduate student when she came to my office. She related that she had pain first in one wrist, but eventually the other wrist hurt, and then the whole arm began to bother her. The pain spread upward to the shoulder and back down again into the hand. Writing, typing and just handling books and papers became intolerable. "When I think back," Margaret remembered, "I was thankful it was in my left hand at the start. But when it was getting uncomfortable in both hands, it became a hardship that kept me from working and threatened my career. My orthopedic doctor diagnosed the condition as carpal tunnel syndrome, a compression of the major nerve that goes from the arm into the hand. His solution was to operate. But surgery meant months of not having the use of my arms and hands, which meant I could not finish my studies. It also required daily physical therapy after the casts were removed and who knows what else! Plus, I did not have good enough health insurance to pay for all of this and my student income was too small to cover the balance. There had to be another way." Margaret's search for an alternative led to acupuncture. It took only three or four treatments for me to reduce the pain substantially in her worse arm and to eliminate it completely in the other. By the end of four or five more sessions, she was back to her normal routine.

Uniformly positive outcomes in my own practice are matched by reports of the success of acupuncture in many countries. Furthermore, these studies show that the treatment works for pain no matter where its location in the body or its original cause. We can see some of these successes in the following studies.

1. Acupuncture and acute and chronic pain: Encouraged by the good results obtained in using acupuncture anesthesia, researchers in Germany started therapeutic acupuncture in outpatient clinics. Acupuncture was regarded as successful when 1) the patient had no complaints at all without medication and 2) there was significant improvement. Treat-

ment for cephalgia (head pain) was successful in 83% of the cases, cervical pain syndromes in 80%, sinusitis in 86%, trigeminal neuralgia in 90%, colitis ulcerosa in 100%, tumor pain in 61%. [2]

In England, the effect of acupuncture was assessed in one hundred and eighty-three patients attending the pain clinic of a cancer hospital. Results were promising, with 82% of the patients obtaining benefit for hours or days. Fifty-three percent obtained significant help, particularly with vascular problems and muscle spasms. The researchers report that acupuncture was significantly helpful with malignant pain problems. [3]

Seventy cases of acute pain were part of a Chinese study on the effects of acupuncture treatment on gastritis, pancreatitis, cholecystitis, rheumatic arthritis, and angina pectoris. Western medical treatment employed antipyretics, analgesics, antispasmodics, and antibiotics. The results were a 94 percent success rate in the acupuncture group compared to 77 percent success rate in the western medicine group. [4]

The long-term effects of acupuncture analgesia are important to pain sufferers. An American study addressed this issue in a six-year follow-up study of 837 patients. These patients were treated in a pain clinic for arthritis, bursitis, tendonitis, low back pain, migraine headaches and trigeminal neuralgia. The results were the majority (73 percent) realized substantial reduction of pain or obtained total pain relief. [5]

2. Acupuncture and temporomandibular joint pain (TMJ): In Finland, twenty-five patients who received acupuncture were compared to twenty-five others who had conventional pain treatment. Results reported that both kinds of treatments produced significant reduction in subjective and clinical symptoms for TMJ dysfunction. Acupuncture was said to be useful in early treatment and worked along with mouth splints to achieve full neuromuscular rehabilitation and to eliminate other contributing factors. [6]

3. Acupuncture and dysmenorrhea (painful menstrual periods): In an American study, women were divided into four groups: a real acupuncture group (given appropriate acupuncture); a placebo acupuncture group (given random point acupuncture); a standard control group (no medical care); and a visitation control group (given monthly conventional care). The results were impressive: ten of the eleven women given real acupuncture showed improvement, while only one of the ten visitation control patients improved. In the placebo acupuncture group the success rate was four out of eleven, and for the standard control group, two of the eleven.[7]

4. Acupuncture and migraine headaches: In a Swedish study,

patients were followed for twelve months after acupuncture therapy. Acupuncture reduced headache attacks considerably for durations of several months or more. In all cases, the sufferers had tried many other therapies before the study. The history of their pain had ranged from seven to forty-eight years. [8]

5. Sports injury and acupuncture: A Swedish study of tennis elbow reported that twenty-one out of thirty-four patients who had received acupuncture were completely free of pain. This was compared to eight out of twenty-six in a control group who recovered after receiving only steroid drugs. The report concluded that acupuncture is a preferred alternative to the use of these drugs. [9]

Acupuncture has proven itself in these and many other recent studies worldwide. German studies concluded that acupuncture should be tried before invasive surgery to cure chronic sinusitis. [10] In a New Zealand study, thirteen patients with neck pain of at least two years' duration participated in acupuncture therapy and reported acupuncture superior to placebo. [11] In a Japanese study of pain from ruptured lumbar disc, excellent success was recorded. [12] Carefully conducted research repeatedly indicates that no matter what part of the body is in pain and no matter what the injury, disease, or malfunction, acupuncture is equally effective or considerably more effective than any other treatment.

Acupuncture is a real alternative for treatment of pain because it works. But there is another, additional consideration when choosing acupuncture: its cost-effectiveness. In most cases, the patient has to absorb the expense of prolonged treatment. It is difficult to make precise comparisons between the cost of acupuncture versus that of conventional medical treatment, but I can give one instructive example. In a recent Australian study, one hundred and forty-five back pain and sciatica cases were treated with acupuncture. The average length of pain had been five years, during which time all the patients had been treated conventionally. The average number of needlings was nine, with a positive rate of effectiveness of 91 percent! [13] We can try to translate this cost of acupuncture treatment into American dollars and cents, as follows: one hundred and forty-five patients multiplied by $40 to $50 (range of treatment fee) multiplied by eight to fifteen treatments gives a range of $46,400 to $119,625 as the total price of acupuncture treatment for all the patients. By comparison, the cost to insurance companies for treatment prior to acupuncture included the following:

- If thirty-six patients had been to chiropractors for about twenty visits at $30 per visit, the total cost is $22,800.
- If twenty-four patients saw physiotherapists three times a week for $50 each time, each for about thirty visits, the total cost is $36,000.
- If surgical procedures were done on eight patients the cost, including any post operative case, could be $41,000.
- Drug costs are difficult to estimate, but if forty-five patients took at least one drug (and some probably two to three drugs several times a day), these 145 patients could spend $72,500 over five years.
- We will have to add the fees for consultations, visits to family doctors and specialists, plus prescriptions for braces, supports, special beds, and so on, at a modest estimated cost of $115,000.

The grand total is $287,300 for the conventional pain treatment for this group of patients. Note that I have excluded losses in income to patients who could not work, and other indirect costs. If these patients had been treated by acupuncture even a few months after the problem appeared, rather than waiting five years, the insurance companies would have saved $156,275 at a minimum and as much as $229,500, a savings of 50 to 80 percent. And if acupuncture therapy had intervened at the onset, at the bedrest stage, the ratio of effectiveness would have been even higher and savings even more impressive.

I will add a final case of evidence. Joan had back pain. Her doctor diagnosed it as sciatica, an inflammation of the sciatic nerve in the lower back and leg. He ordered her to go to bed for six weeks, to do no work at all, and to keep all basic activities to a minimum. She was told that if this did not help, another six weeks of bedrest would be needed. Then if there was still no progress, he would consider surgery. In desperation at the prospect of at least three months of inactivity, and perhaps surgery in addition, she chose to try acupuncture. After five treatments, her pain vanished, and she has been pain-free for the last three years.

Most back pain sufferers do not undergo surgery. For most cases like Joan's, the standard orthopedic advice is bedrest, pain medication, physical therapy, or some combination of these. But prolonged bedrest can slow healing. Pain medication may or may not work, does not cure, and can be habit forming.

In the United States, an enormous amount of money is spent annually on treatment for pain. In addition, a vast amount of money is lost in poor work performance and lost work hours. The loss in strained relationships and general unhappiness is incalculable. Is it any wonder that for many pain sufferers acupuncture has become a viable alternative to conventional treatments? Even when the patient continues a standard route like physical therapy or chiropractic adjustment, acupuncture is beneficial in accelerating recovery. Research results, my own clinical experience, simple economics, and a bit of common sense all point to acupuncture as the first offense against debilitating pain.

NOTES

1. Edgar Berman, *The Solid Gold Stethoscope,* New York: Wiley, 1976, 122.
2. M. V. Fisher. "Acupuncture Therapy in the Outpatient Department of the Heidelberg University Clinic." *Anaesthetist* 31(1):25-32, 1982.
3. J. Filshie, D. Redman. *International Medical Acupuncture Conference*, London, May 4-8, 1986. Meeting paper.
4. Qi Muzhen, et al. "Acute Pain Treated by Acupuncture." *Chinese Acupuncture and Moxibustion.* 6 (2):21-22, 1986.
5. Pang L. Man, and T. L. Ning. "Acupuncture Treatment for Chronic Pain: A Six-Year Follow-up Study." *American Journal of Acupuncture.* 10 (2):165-166, 1982.
6. A. M. Raustia, et al. "The Alternative Treatment of Temperomandibular Joint (TMJ) Dysfunction with Acupuncture." *First Theoretical-Practical International Seminar of Complementary Techniques*, Oct. 23-25, 1987. Meeting paper.
7. J. M. Helms. "Acupuncture for the Management of Primary Dysmenorrhea." *Obstetrics and Gynecology.* 69 (1):51-56, 1987.
8. J. Boivie, G. Brattberg. "An Evaluation of Acupuncture Treatment for Migraine." *Acta Neurology Scandinavia.* 69 (S-98):268-269, 1984.
9. G. Brattberg. "Acupuncture therapy for Tennis Elbow." *Pain.* 16 (3):285-288, 1983.
10. R. Pothmann, H. L. Yeh. "Effects of Treatment with Antibiotics, Laser, and Acupuncture upon Chronic Maxillary Sinusits in Children." *American Journal of Chinese Medicine.* 10 (1-4):55-58, 1982.
11. J. B. Petrie, G. B. Langley. "Acupuncture in Treatment of Chronic Cervical Pain: A Pilot Study." *Clinical and Experimental Rheumatology.* 1 (4):333-335, 1983.
12. T. Maruyama. "Acupuncture Treatment for Ruptured Lumbar Disc

II." *Journal of the Japan Society of Acupuncture.* 33 (4):375-382, 1984.
13. G. Mendelson, et al. "Acupuncture Treatment of Chronic Back Pain: A Double-Blind Placebo-Controlled Trial." *American Journal of Medicine.* 74 (1):49-55, 1983.

REFERENCES

Detailed strategies and applications of Traditional Chinese Medicine and pain relief can be found in L. Chaitow, *The Acupuncture Treatment of Pain* (1983) and in P. E. Baldry, *Acupuncture, Trigger Points and Musculoskeletal Pain* (1989).

Chapter 6

ACUPUNCTURE ANESTHESIA

Until the late 1950s Chinese doctors used Western drugs and procedures to induce general anesthesia during surgery. The Cultural Revolution changed this approach. First, a dangerous shortage of modern medical facilities and personnel made it urgent that they find readily available alternatives. Second, the Chinese government wished to favor Chinese over Western practices for ideological reasons—to show that Eastern ways were equal to or better than Western ways. Practitioners of the ancient medical arts still existed and were ready to teach the nearly forgotten skills. So Chinese physicians began to study the great storehouse of knowledge that is Traditional Chinese Medicine and to adapt its techniques to modern needs. They soon discovered that acupuncture enabled them to make incisions painlessly while their patients remained fully conscious.

In the beginning, acupuncture was used for minor operations such as tonsillectomies and dental surgery. By the mid-1970s more than 400,000 Chinese patients had received acupuncture anesthesia. Today acupuncture is employed in more than two hundred different surgical procedures, from mild to serious cases, from infants to octogenarians.

Acupuncture anesthesia is administered by inserting a few needles into either the external ear or the body. The acupuncturist-anesthetist then connects the head or blunt end of the needles to a low-voltage electric stimulating device. Within approximately fifteen to forty-five minutes the patient's awareness of pain sensation is reduced enough to allow the surgeon to proceed. The mechanism of pain reduction appears to be transmission of impulses through hormones and neurotransmitters. Experiments on animals show that when cerebral fluid from needled animals is transferred to others that have not been needled, the analgesic effects still take place. In humans, acupuncture analgesia lasts up to twenty hours after the removal of needles.

It is difficult to compare Chinese and Western methods of anesthesia. Chinese practices do not lend themselves to the same conceptual categories as those in the West. With Western methods, the patient awakens in the postoperative ward with no recollection of either pain or the surgery; he has been completely anesthetized. In the Chinese version, only analgesia—pain reduction—has taken place, so that the term anesthesia does not fit.

Acupuncture anesthesia does not "knock out" the patient, as do conventional drugs. Instead, it raises the patient's overall pain threshold— the level at which one begins to feel pain—specifically at the locale of the surgery. The patient does remain capable of feeling other stimuli, such as temperature changes, pressure, and touch. He can also see, hear, speak, and control body motion thoughout the operation.

Moreover, there is no clear distinction between local and general anesthesia in the Chinese method. Acupuncture analgesia, with its intense sensory inputs, activates special areas in the brain, which in turn inhibits pain impulses from various body parts. Thus, conceivably, acupuncture stimulation at a point such as the wrist can kill pain in the chest.

Acupuncture anesthesia offers major advantages that drug anesthesia cannot claim. Because the patient is fully conscious, he can help the surgeon monitor the work while it is in progress and make subtle adjustments in the procedure. In extremely delicate and precise undertakings, such as the removal of the thyroid gland, the surgeon can ask the patient to speak, ensuring that he does no damage to the patient's vocal functions. In orthopedic work, such as hand surgery, acupuncture anesthesia lets the patient move his fingers, thus assisting the surgeon in the safe repair of injured areas. Rather than remaining passive and unconscious, the patient can cooperate in his treatment and contribute significantly to the success of the surgery.

Acupuncture has further advantages over drug anesthesia. Blood pressure, pulse rate, and respiration remain stable and normal; they do not have to be artificially maintained with the aid of complex machinery. Because the length of time spent in surgery is significantly less, the patient loses less blood and the wound heals faster. Patients usually do not suffer the postsurgical complications of nausea and vomiting, nor are they dehydrated. The generalized raising of the pain threshold continues for a time after the surgery, so that patients request postsurgical painkillers in only small quantities, if at all. Following many kinds of operations, patients may take a long while to recover from the anesthetic drugs themselves; with acupuncture, surgical recovery is remarkably fast. They can move about on their own and take nourishment as soon as the needles are removed, if the surgery has been of such a nature to permit these activities.

Like other applications of acupuncture, its use as anesthesia is continually being refined. With operating room experience, it has been possible to reduce the total number of needles used and to isolate specific points in order to achieve the desired effects. In lung surgery, for example, researchers analyzed the results of three hundred operations and some twenty different combinations of points in an attempt to locate the single most effective combination. These research findings are now used routinely. One needle point prevents difficulty in breathing once the chest cavity has been opened. A second point is needled to block the pain of the surgery.

At the Seventh World Congress of Anesthesiologists held in Hamburg, Germany, in 1980, seventeen scientific papers on electroacupuncture were presented. One of the largest research projects reported on was conducted in West Germany. In eight hundred cases of coronary bypass and aortic valve replacement procedures, acupuncture was tested against conventional narcotic anesthesia. A standard criterion of evaluation was used to measure the adequacy of analgesia in either case: the dose of narcotics administered during surgery. Patients not receiving acupuncture required significantly greater amounts of blood thinners and narcotics. Fewer blood thinners were needed for acupuncture subjects because a specific point was needled in the arm to produce a necessary drop in blood pressure, heart rate, and arterial pressure. The postoperative condition of the acupuncture group was markedly better than that of the control group patients: immediately after surgery 70 percent of the acupuncture patients could be extubated (have the air tubes inserted down the throat removed), while only 23 percent of the control group could tolerate the withdrawal of tubes. During the first hours just after surgery, acupuncture patients needed less postoperative morphine than control patients, probably because of the "endorphin high" that acupuncture produced. The advantage of using acupuncture as a surgical anesthesia could not be more conclusively demonstrated.

Acupuncture anesthesia is being used all over the world. Clinical and experimental research has shown that it can be a better choice in many procedures where conventional methods are used. For example:

- Tooth extractions (Japan): Coupled with premedication of D-phenylaniline, acupuncture gave good results. Premedication enhances analgesic effects, results in no pain, and obviates the need for supplementary anesthesia.[1]
- Urological surgery (Holland): Acupuncture entirely replaced standard drug use in operations lasting three to four hours.[2]
- Splenectomy (China): In a study of sixty-four cases of spleen removal, a 98 percent success rate was reported.[3]
- Upper gastrointestinal endoscopy (Nigeria): The overall success rate was 88 percent, about the same as for conventional methods.[4]
- Caesarean section (China): A comparison was done of six hundred and sixty-four cases with acupuncture to two hundred and thirty-seven under epidural anesthesia. With acupuncture, changes in blood pressure and pulse were negligible, less blood loss occurred, and the analgesic effect was satisfactory. No postoperative complications occurred, and there was a better return of gastrointestinal function with acupuncture than with epidural anesthesia.[5]
- Radiosurgery for oral neoplasms (Italy): The monitoring of twelve patients who underwent the removal of cancerous masses showed acupuncture to have remarkable advantages over either local or general anesthesia. Local anesthesia usually produces edema and requires tubes in the nose. Acupuncture gives excellent analgesia and does not cause local complications as do conventional techniques.[6]
- Abdominal operations (China): A study focused on one thousand, one hundred and twenty patients who had acupuncture for abdominal surgery. The success rate was 99 percent.[7]

If you are not too squeamish to observe the surgical removal of a man's brain tumor under acupuncture, come with me into the operating room.

The fully conscious patient is wheeled in and gently transferred to the operating table. He is thin, slightly taller than average, 38 years old. Six months ago, he suffered the onset of severe convulsions. Since then, he has experienced loss of muscle tone in his left arm and leg, and his left hand and foot are almost completely paralyzed. If the brain tumor is not removed and it continues to grow, it will cause general paralysis, then death. There is a risk because necessary surgery can damage healthy brain tissue. So the medical team and the patient have agreed that acupuncture will be the anesthesia to allow the patient to remain conscious and responsive during the procedure.

The acupuncturist begins by inserting five needles in the patient's external ear, hands, and legs and then couples electrical leads to the needles' blunt ends. The points will provide intense stimulation to counteract the pain that would otherwise accompany the first stage of surgery— cutting the scalp. The acupuncturist waits twenty minutes to allow needles to effect the desired chemical changes. He then tests for pain, probing and questioning. The patient says that all is well, although he is apprehensive.

During the drilling and sawing, the patient is awake and alert but relaxed. Having a conscious patient can make the surgeon's work easier. Although the surgical team operates on the patient's exposed brain with precision and speed, the patient is asked to move his limbs, fingers and toes—body parts that up until now have been paralyzed. He is also asked to blink and to speak. By enlisting the patient's cooperation, the surgeon can be more exact.

The surgeon is now satisfied that he has removed all of the tumor and that no loss of motor abilities has taken place. He cleanses the wound, closes it, and sutures the scalp. Following the procedure intensely, the acupuncturist has increased electrical stimulation as required to maintain analgesic reaction.

The team stands back while the acupuncturist removes his needles. The patient is helped to sit up on the edge of the operating table. He smiles and jokes with the doctor and nurses. When offered a glass of orange juice, he drinks it eagerly. Accompanied by his nurses, he walks back to his hospital bed. After a short recuperation period, he will return home and will soon be back at his job—experiencing a speedy recovery from an illness that had incapacitated him for many months.

NOTES

1.   M. Hyodo, et al. "Acupuncture Anesthesia with D-Phenylalanine." *Journal of the Japan Society of Acupuncture and Moxibustion.* 31 (2):136-139, 1981.
2.   H. G. Kho, et al. "Acupuncture Anesthesia in Urologic Surgery: A Pilot Study." *Deutsche Zeitschrift fur Akupunktur.* 30 (3):60-64, 1987.
3.   Hu Limei. "Clinical Observations of 64 Splenectomies Under Acupuncture Anesthesia." *Chinese Acupuncture and Moxibustion.* 7 (3):23-24, 1987.
4.   J.O.A. Sodipo, T.A.J. Ogunbiyi. "Acupuncture Analgesia for Upper Gastrointestinal Endoscopy: A Lagos Experience." *American Journal of Chinese Medicine.* 9 (2):171-173, 1981.
5.   Acupuncture Anesthesia Group. "Caesarean Section Under Acupuncture Anesthesia." *Chinese Acupuncture and Moxibustion.* 3 (5):13-15, 1983.
6.   N. Mortellaro, et al. "Acupuncture Analgesia in Radiosurgical Treatment for Oral Cavity Neoplasm." *International Medical Acupuncture Conference*: London, May 4-8, 1986. Meeting paper.
7.   Qin Xueli. "Abdominal Operations Performed Under Acupuncture Anesthesia Using the Du Channel: A Report of 1,120 Cases." *Chinese Acupuncture and Moxibustion.* 6 (4):22-24, 1986.

REFERENCES

More information on acupuncture anesthesia can be found in J. O'Connor and D. Bensky, trans. and eds., *Acupuncture: A Comprehensive Text* (1981).

Chapter 7

SCALP AND EAR ACUPUNCTURE: THE REPAIR OF THE BRAIN AND NERVOUS SYSTEM

Within your brain lies a marvelous control center of sensory and motor faculties. This is the brain's cerebral cortex, the last organ to fully develop in the embryo, and the most evolved in its capacity to direct the multitude of body processes. Divided into two hemispheres of equal size, the cerebral cortex is only 2 or 3 millimeters thick. This part of the brain is subdivided into many discrete sections, each of which relays information and commands to all parts of the body.

When damage occurs in certain parts of this cortex, the result could be corresponding loss of control over voluntary movements in a specific limb. For example, an injury to the back of the cortex can result in paresthesia (a loss in the ability to sense and analyze heat, touch, and pain). If injury occurs to the front of the cortex, paralysis in one or more parts of the body may follow. Midarea trauma can cause tinnitus (ringing in the ear), vertigo, loss of equilibrium, and impaired hearing.

Other cortex areas analyze and then execute the movements required for delicate work, such as the ability to sew. An example is the "Broca area," named after the French surgeon Paul Broca. Here lies control of all the muscles of the mouth, tongue, pharynx, and larynx. A dysfunction or injury here causes motor aphasia (the inability to speak).

Visualization, which requires organizing and relating extremely complex sensations—color, size, perspective, and distance—can be impaired when brain tissue is damaged or diseased. If this part of the brain suffers pathology, patients may experience visual hallucinations, confusion, and other specific motor disturbances as well as decreased muscle tone.

The brain's interior houses the internal capsule, a relay station of complex fibers radiating out to the cortex. These fibers relay the entire body's sensory data up and down the spinal column. Injury to these fibers causes paralysis in one or both sides of the body.

At the back of the brain is the cerebellum, which controls equilibrium and coordination. Injury to the cerebellum causes ataxia (loss of muscle coordination in the limbs). Thus, a cerebral hemorrhage (bleeding in the head), inflammation, or head trauma, will often cause loss of balance and poor hand-to-eye coordination.

After the Chinese Revolution, researchers devoted themselves to integrating Traditional Medicine and modern Western science, putting acupuncture's elegant simplicity to work on "incurable" brain disorders. One process they developed is scalp acupuncture, which was initially used to treat cerebral thrombosis (obstruction of blood supply to the brain), comatose cerebral hemorrhage (bleeding in the brain area with accompanying unconsciousness), and acute cranial trauma. Later experimentation and advances centered on cranial inflammations, which are common to diseases such as choreas and paralysis agitans (diseases of the nervous system characterized by jerky, involuntary movements), paralysis with muscular atrophy (wasting away), sclerosis (hardening of tissue), and neuralgia (pain).

Western treatments of surgery, extensive physical therapy, and rehabilitation are lengthy and complicated. Even with this large inventory of conventional techniques, brain injury does not respond well to intervention. Regaining the use of limbs and restoring manual dexterity are especially problematic. Scalp acupuncture, by contrast, especially if begun within a few weeks after the onset of injury, is effective in many cases in which patients would otherwise have spent the rest of their lives in a wheelchair or bed.

Needling is applied directly to the surface of the head. A system has been precisely mapped out that correlates placement of the needle directly over the area of the underlying brain that corresponds to the lost or impaired body function. For instance, in treating loss of speech, we needle the scalp directly over the Broca area. If the problem is lower limb paralysis, we needle along a line parallel to the front-to-back head midline motor area controlling the legs.

Needle insertion is made just under the skin at an angle of fifteen degrees to the scalp, to a depth of one-fourth to one half-inch. The patient feels little pain. Unless both limbs are affected, the side opposite the malfunctioning limb is needled. The hair is not shaved or cut. Needles remain in place for about twenty minutes, and then are withdrawn painlessly. Treatments are repeated at intervals of two to three times a week, sometimes for several months, until the desired result is achieved. The program is intensive, not unlike a physical therapy rehabilitation program.

Many Chinese studies report scalp acupuncture can be remarkably successful. In a twenty-six patient study of sequelae of cerebrovascular accident or cerebral injury, needling on the scalp provided multiple benefits. Acupuncture improved microcirculation, promoted the resolution of blood stasis, and alleviated anoxia or lack of oxygen of the brain tissue. Acupuncture reduced blood pressure and lowered agglutinating factors of the blood, reducing its viscosity and preventing the formation of microemboli. In addition, the scalp areas selected for acupuncture were related to functional areas of the cerebral cortex and therefore could promote recovery of injured brain tissue.[1]

Researchers have found no significant relationship between age of patients and success of treatment. A positive correlation did exist between onset of treatment and treatment outcome. If acupuncture was undertaken within ten days of the onset of the condition, results were positive for 57 percent of the patients. When treatment was given between eleven days and three months after onset, the success rate dropped to 37 percent. After four to six months following injury, acupuncture worked for only 27 percent. The sooner the treatment, the better the chances of recovery. [2]

Another study of one hundred and forty-three cases of cerebroparalysis in children and adults was conducted for scalp areas correlating to motor, speech, visual, and memory functions. The results suggest that many cases may be cured.[3]

One two-year research project consisted of ninety-two cases of cerebral hemorrhage. The courses of illness ranged from one to six days. Six of the patients were in deep coma, eight in moderate coma, and fifteen were mildly comatose. The cases were randomly divided into two groups of forty-six cases each: one for acupuncture treatment, and one for control. Patients were needled once daily. The results showed that the rate of cure reached fifty percent with acupuncture treatment. There was recovery of consciousness and speech and motor function of the limbs. [4]

Pioneering scalp acupuncture therapy at first concentrated on brain injury. Gradually, with experience, its use was expanded to treat other long-term diseases, such as encephalitis (brain inflammation), the choreas, migraine headache, Parkinson's disease, and Menière's syndrome (severe dizziness and nausea). Success with these early applications encouraged practitioners to extend the field still further. Scalp acupuncture has also proved effective in treating torticolis (a fixed twisting of the neck), arthritis, back and limb pain, childhood bedwetting, and adult incontinence.

In clinical work from China, acupuncture's effectiveness is exciting. A 54-year-old male brickmaker was brought to the hospital with paralysis to the right side of his body, elevated blood pressure, tongue deviation to the right side, complete paralysis of the right leg, and partial paralysis of the right arm. He was diagnosed with cerebral thrombosis. As soon as he was stabilized, his doctors began scalp needling of the appropriate left motor and sensory stimulation areas. After five treatments, he regained use of both his right arm and leg. One year later, he was in normal control of all his limbs and in a good state of mind. He had also returned to work.

A second case, a 24-year-old laborer, was accidentally hit on the head and had been unconscious for seven days. Upon regaining consciousness, he had complete paralysis of the right arm and loss of speech. On the eleventh day after injury, his doctors began scalp acupuncture. After nineteen treatments, the patient left the hospital speaking fluently, experienced no further dizziness or headaches, and had command over the use of his arm. A year later, he still showed no aftereffects from the accident.

A third case was a 2-year-old girl who developed a high fever and went into a coma that lasted two weeks. The fever persisted, accompanied by convulsion. She went blind and was paralyzed in all limbs. Her neck was very weak and could not support her head. After five straight days of acupuncture she could see. With twenty days of needling, she began to use her arms and legs. Following additional treatments, she stood up. At her first year's follow-up examination, she was in good health.

A 15-year-old girl diagnosed with chorea had symptoms of involuntary movement, spastic jerking, grimacing, and protruding tongue. Eventually she could neither sit still nor walk. Her doctors began daily scalp needling that continued for two weeks. A month later the agitation in her limbs was gone, and she was released from the hospital. A year later she was perfectly fit and had returned to school and a normal daily routine.

I have used scalp acupuncture to treat some unusual cases. One involved an older man who started treatment for shaking. He had been to several neurologists who diagnosed Parkinson's disease. But he did not respond to the usually prescribed medication. One neurologist simply told him it was hereditary. The patient said that many of the men in his family shook, but not all of them were afflicted in the same way; his father's hands shook, his grandfather's head and hands shook, his own head and hands shook.

In the beginning, his wife paid for sessions by writing out the checks. On the last treatment, he asked for the checkbook. With a grand flourish of his hand, he took up a pen to write out the check, something he had been unable to do for years.

Another interesting case was that of a woman who had been diagnosed with postpolio syndrome. The polio she had had as a child seemed to have been completely cured. Now in her late 40s, she had started feeling pain in all of her limbs. Her muscle tone was wasting, and she was unable to use her limbs. She had steadily declined until she had to remain in bed for many days and use a walker when she felt strong enough to move around.

After examining her, I decided to try scalp acupuncture; this method allowed me to work on all four limbs at each treatment session. She responded very well. Each successive treatment brought a lessening of pain and greater mobility. After we finished the original series of ten weekly treatments, she could walk unaided and could be active most days and even do some housework. She looked like a different person.

When the central nervous system is injured, motor responses and capacities close down. For instance, in polio (anterior horn poliomyelitis), there may be hemorrhaging, infiltration of the affected area by foreign cells, inflammation, blockage of nutrients, and grave damage to the central nervous system cells themselves. All of these pathologies can lead to blocking of the command impulses between the brain and body parts, closing the gateway of communication between them. This blocking is the immediate cause of paralysis. Spinal cord nerve cells stop working. Some acupuncture theorists say that needling can force the neurons into transmitting again, even after a long passage of time, by creating a passage between the damaged and undamaged parts of the spinal cord and brain. This passage may open when acupuncture promotes the body's production of certain natural chemical and hormonal agents in formerly inactive neurons.

The mechanics governing motor control are a complicated closed-loop system that can be impaired or shut off completely if neurons in the spinal cord cannot communicate sensations to the brain or if the brain cannot transmit its wishes to the appropriate part of the body. Acupuncture reopens these gates and restores the lines of communication between the brain and the body by stimulating chemical and electrical changes in the nerve cells. Another possibility advanced by researchers is that of acupuncture's ability to reroute around inactive neurons and tap into the vast neuron pools lying dormant behind the inactive ones.

Practitioners recommend that acupuncture be used in treating all paralytic disorders. If acupuncture is going to work at all, it begins showing positive signs early on. One clinical study testing speed of recovery in fifty-three ataxia (defective muscular coordination) cases showed improvement within ten days of daily treatment. In follow-up evaluation of discharged patients, the evidence showed that the improvements were permanent.

The aurical, or external ear, has been another subject of intensive research in China. Study of the aurical has led to the discovery and mapping of over two hundred points. The uses of ear acupuncture in treating disease are almost limitless. The ear is also an appropriate site for administering acupuncture anesthesia during surgical and dental treatments and for treating substance abuse.

Ancient documents and lore contain many sophisticated guides to treatment of human maladies through the external ear. Some of these documents deal with diagnosis by ear examination and discuss numerous types of treatment, such as pricking and drawing blood from an area and ear massage techniques. In ancient Egypt, women used needling as a contraceptive. Arabs, Gypsies, Hindus, and even Europeans needled a point on the ear lobe to correct eye problems. Special earrings were worn to provide continuous stimulation to the brain to restore vision. Hippocrates wrote of a treatment for male impotence which involved needling the ear.

The Arabs, familiar with acupuncture from the thirteenth century, cauterized specific points on the ear to ameliorate sciatica or pain in the lower back and legs.

The ancients knew that the external ear has a rich supply of nerves and blood vessels that communicate with the major areas of the brain. Modern pathology uses the ear in a diagnostic way, looking for discolorations, hypersensitivity, scars, and texture changes that show up in the ear over internal organ points.

Present-day knowledge and theory regarding the ear's relationship to the rest of the body originated in the work of Chinese practitioners. The method of using the ear as a diagnostic and therapeutic tool was developed in 1957 by Dr. Paul Nogier of Lyon, France. He theorized that the ear can be "read," providing an assessment of the state of health of the entire body. He superimposed a body upside down on the ear, so that the head corresponds to the lobe, the internal organs appear in the internal cavities, and the spinal cord is represented by the protruding spine of the ear.

In order to evaluate his theory, Dr. Nogier did extensive testing on skin impedance and resistance, which he measured by electrical readings on the ear's surface. He measured sensitivity to mechanical stimulation, such as touching points with a probe and heat application. He called the ear the "gateway to the body."

Dr. Nogier's research has been replicated in studies by Dr. Yoshiaki Omura. In one study of one hundred volunteers, he accurately diagnosed 55 percent of the patients' diseases just through ear examination, establishing a better track record than that of the average Western practitioner. With no prior knowledge of the patients' medical histories or current states of health, he made accurate diagnoses by ear reading alone. He found, for example, that deep grooves in the lower part of the ear lobe had abnormally low electrical resistance and indicated cardiovascular disease. These diseases often appear among subjects with hypertension, myocardial infarction (heart attack), and angina pectoris (blood supply blockage to the heart) in middle-aged and older people.[5]

Ear diagnosis and treatment are included in many practitioners' standard treatment plans. Treatment can focus on ear points alone or on ear points in conjunction with body points. Techniques include electrical stimulation of the needles and tiny needles left on the ear point for short periods of time to provide continued stimulation. Ion-sphere pellets or magnets can be taped to the points to provide low-level continuous treatment.

Scalp and ear techniques have been used to reverse many serious illnesses. Among these illnesses are disorders of the brain and central nervous system that, up to now, have been resistant to correction. Traditional Chinese Medicine has been combined with Western science in both diagnostic and therapeutic use to the enrichment of both. We can expect many new discoveries from the cross-fertilization.

NOTES

1.   Ji Nan, et al. "A Study on the Mechanism of Acupuncture Therapy in the Treatment of Sequelae of Cerebrovascular Accident or Cerebral Injury." *Journal of Traditional Chinese Medicine.* 7 (3):165-168, 1987.
2.   Dong Guirong, et al. "Clinical Observation on Treatment of 48 Cases of Acute Cerebral Hemorrhage by Scalp Acupuncture." *Chinese Acupuncture and Moxibustion.* 10 (91):19-20, 1990.
3.   Lin Hsio-Chien. "A Study of the Clinical Efficacy of the New Areas—Silent Areas—in Scalp Acupuncture." *Fourth International Congress of Chinese Medicine*, San Francisco, July 29-31, 1988. Meeting paper.
4.   Li Dingming, et al. "Clinical Observation on Acupuncture Therapy for Cerebral Hemorrhage." *Journal of Traditional Chinese Medicine.* 9(1):9-13, 1989.
5.   Yoshiaki Omura, *Acupuncture Medicine.* Tokyo: Japan Publications, 1982, 249.

REFERENCES

A general introduction to these subjects can be found in M. Wexu *The Ear: Gateway to Balancing the Body* (1982). Information on newer techniques and advances such as scalp acupuncture appears in Y. Omura, *Acupuncture Medicine* (1982).

Chapter 8

REPAIR OF ORTHOPEDIC INJURY: CHINESE HIT MEDICINE

"Hit Medicine" was developed centuries ago in China to treat muscular and skeletal damage suffered in martial arts and fighting. Today, Hit Medicine provides relief from any sort of trauma, treats pain and swelling, and promotes rapid healing and early recovery of the use of the injured body part. In my practice I have successfully used traditional Hit Medicine for both sport-related injuries and orthopedic damage suffered in my patients' daily lives.

When Helen fell from a ladder, she hobbled to her health care clinic. Her knee was painful, swollen, and discolored. An orthopedic doctor prescribed an Ace bandage, crutches, and bedrest. He said he would take X-rays when the swelling subsided. On her way home, still in pain, she remembered me and stopped to call from a pay telephone. A year before, she had been helped dramatically when I acupunctured her for hand, wrist, and arm pain diagnosed as carpal tunnel syndrome. I asked her to come to my office immediately, and we started a therapy program of needling, heat and massage.

One week and three treatments rid the area of swelling, bruising, and pain. But the knee did not feel right to her. We agreed that she should return to the clinic for an X-ray. The picture showed a dislocated kneecap. Once again, a doctor prescribed crutches and two to three weeks of bedrest. This time she did not hesitate to call me and came directly to my office. I began using a point prescription that one of my teachers, Dr. James So, had developed for just such injuries. After four treatments, the kneecap gradually returned to a normal position. She was pain-free and back to work in about a quarter of the time it would have taken had she followed her doctor's advice.

Bob fell on his left side while doing carpentry and landed heavily on his knee. As the day wore on, the knee swelled to twice its normal size and hurt terribly. His wife drove him to an emergency room where a doctor took X-rays and diagnosed a case of fluid on the knee. He ordered Bob to stay off the leg and prescribed pain medication.

Bob stayed home in his easy chair and took his painkillers dutifully. After several days with no improvement, he began to get edgy; as a self-employed worker, he was losing time and money. He cast about for alternatives to the treatment he was receiving and remembered having read about acupuncture treatment for pain. He telephoned me, and I arranged an evening visit to his home. I encircled his kneecap with needles, heating some of them with an herb stick. That night he experienced unusual sensations in his knee and leg, "as if water were running up and down." He slept well, and the next morning the swelling was visibly reduced and his pain was almost gone. One more session restored his knee to normal size. We decided that he could return to work on a limited basis. He received a final treatment, strengthening the knee and leg.

Lucy was 79 years old when she first came for treatment. She had a swollen, tender foot, although she could not remember hurting it. An orthopedic physician initially diagnosed osteoporosis, a bone disease common among the elderly. But X-rays contradicted that diagnosis, so the next guess was that she had torn some ligaments. She was told to bandage the foot and ankle, use crutches, stay off the foot completely, and take prescription drugs for pain relief.

Lucy found it hard to follow the advice. She could not tolerate the side effects of the pain medication, and because she lived alone, she had to move around to take care of herself. She feared a prolonged recovery. She followed her doctor's orders for about a week. When there was no noticeable improvement, she made an appointment for acupuncture.

Three treatments did the trick. Her pain disappeared, and her foot returned to normal size.

Living and working in Vermont was Tim's dream come true until he shattered his ankle in a fall. He managed to drive himself to an emergency clinic. The break was severe enough to require surgery, and he was told that a long recuperation would be necessary. While he was still in the orthopedic doctor's office, Tim asked to use the telephone and called to ask my opinion. I suggested that if the area could be splinted after surgery, I could work on it then.

Tim underwent surgery and was told that he would be unable to walk or work for seven months. He would need extensive physical therapy. He arranged to be moved down to Boston for treatment and nursing care. I made several home visits until he was able to move around on crutches. I worked on the ankle twice a week, supplementing needling with herbal medicines. Within two months he could put weight on the foot and walk with a cane. The accident happened in late January; Tim had the surgery in early February; and he was walking normally in April. When he reported for the physical therapy prescribed by his doctor, the therapist's evaluation showed there was nothing to work on. She did see him once to demonstrate some exercises he could do on his own. By June, he was back to work on his construction job.

People who follow a sport or exercise program often hurt themselves badly enough to need treatment. I have treated body builders with aching knees, backs, and shoulders. I have worked with amateur and professional athletes, as well as with teachers and students. When they hurt, they want help that works.

An instructor of Thai boxing once sought my assistance for a muscle tear in his leg. This injury had interrupted Roger's teaching and training. He had consulted with an orthopedist and a neurologist, both of whom advised complete rest but prescribed no other treatment. If the leg did not quickly recover, one said, surgery would have to be performed. Roger came to me, and I gave him a needling treatment and herbal ointment to apply. We repeated the procedure two days later. Because the injury was recent and the man was physically fit, I expected the leg to respond quickly. He reported dramatic reduction in swelling and pain after the first treatment. We had a third session a week later. He was soon back with his students, having missed only two weeks of work.

Many people ask about the use of acupuncture on tennis elbow. Some of these inquiries come from tennis players themselves, and some come from people who have injured themselves through routine wear and tear of the arm. One interesting case was presented to me about six years ago. I was a guest at a gathering of health care practitioners and met a physician who was an ardent tennis player. He half-jokingly challenged me to tell him what acupuncture could do for his tennis elbow. I responded by asking him to tell me the history of his condition. He said that the problem was many months old, and at first he'd treated it himself with medicines. When there was no improvement, he received cortisone injections from an orthopedist. Next, he began a program of physical therapy several times a week which he had attended for the last three months. Thus far, nothing had helped.

I told him that acupuncture relieves nine out of ten cases like his and added that since he had exhausted all his conventional options, he could make an appointment with me for treatment. The very next week we began. I gave his elbow five treatments very close together in time and advised that he suspend exercise and tennis for awhile. In the month that followed, he rested the arm and experienced no pain or further swelling. Then he began to play in very short easy sessions without discomfort. He gradually returned to his former regimen of three vigorous tennis matches a week. Last year my physician-patient called to report another bothersome tendonitis (inflammation of the tendon) and asked me to treat it. Once a skeptic, he now told me that he would skip injections and physical therapy in favor of acupuncture, which he knew would work! This time he was back on the tennis court after just four treatments.

Contrast the rapid recoveries of Bob, Helen, Lucy, Tim and others with the drawn-out, uncomfortable, and painful healing process each would have experienced with Western orthopedic medicine. The conventional route entails periods of complete inactivity, followed by weeks or months of physical therapy, two or three times a week. Finally, there is the worry about one's job and fear that the injured area will never again be the same.

What can you do if you or someone close to you has an accident? First-aid may be called for: cleaning the wound, stopping blood flow if necessary, and immobilizing the area with a temporary splint or cast. Setting bones, suturing wounds, and administering antibiotics are all early measures that Western medicine performs very well. If there is any doubt about the nature and extent of the injury, X-rays can be taken for evaluation and diagnosis. After these standard diagnostic procedures have been performed, it is time for Traditional Chinese Medicine to step in to help the body heal itself.

Treatment for injuries can begin immediately. Pain relief and reduction of swelling come first. When there are bruises, contusions, and broken blood vessels, the acupuncturist works on dispersing this coagulated blood. We use needling techniques at precisely indicated locations and administer herbal plasters and medicines to speed up the healing process. When appropriate, we use massage. Acupuncture is great for treating sprains and damage to muscle tissue, tendons, ligaments, and joint capsules—particularly if it is undertaken soon after the accident.

Needling has multiple benefits. First, needling increases the circulation of the blood. This increase in circulation is seen in the slight reddening of the skin around the needle as it sits in the point and in the rise in skin temperature just after needling. By increased circulation through a traumatized area, dead and coagulated cells are cleansed away and healing is accelerated. Studies show that the flow of blood to injured limbs is greatly impaired when the blood supply is blocked by vessel paralysis, spasm, or contraction. Almost immediately, needling brings a much-needed supply of both white blood cells to cleanse and fight possible infection and red blood cells to generate new tissue growth.

Second, needling decreases muscle tension and the tightness of connective tissue. Spasms and contractions can be relieved without the use of drugs. A kind of natural "splinting" takes place following an injury— a stiffening of surrounding tissue. This splinting is beneficial at an early stage but often impedes healing if it persists. Acupuncture helps to relax this reflex. Indeed, some Western neurologists "dry needle" or insert an empty hypodermic needle for just this purpose. The goal is to break up muscle congestion, and whether or not they wish to admit it, these doctors are, in fact, practicing acupuncture.

Third, acupuncture stimulates positive chemical changes in the body. Specific neurotransmitters, among them endorphins and enkephalins, elevate concentrations of chemicals in the brain and thus raise the threshold of pain. Evidence shows that needling also produces hormonal chemicals. These chemicals include a natural cortisol (similar to steroid cortisone drugs), magnesium ions, and adrenocorticotropic hormone. This last chemical stimulates adrenal glands to resolve the stress of trauma.

Even when treatment is postponed for a time, needling promotes healing. This often happens when patients come to acupuncture after having tried other therapies without result. I have treated cases of torn ligament and tendon, tennis elbow, injured muscles, and damaged knees weeks and even months after the injury occurred. I have also reversed limb atrophy caused by long immobility in casts.

Western medicine treats fractures routinely. Broken bones do need to be set and protected for a time. The Chinese, however, have made improvements on the conventional plaster cast; they use flexible bamboo splints and padded supports that allow the acupuncturist to work on the injured area immediately. Many thousands of broken bones have been set in this manner in the orthopedic hospitals of China, and the healing time has been cut in half. Moreover, this treatment has none of the usual side effects of casts such as deep muscle spasm, atrophy, and weakness. Sometimes physical therapy is not even needed. In my practice, I have worked on breaks for which casts are not usually applied, such as fractured noses, ribs, and toes. Again, with acupuncture and herbs, these heal in about half the time taken by conventional treatment.

Though prolonged bedrest may appeal to a person who has just suffered a trauma, after one week of immobility, the body begins to fall into dilapidation like a vacant house. Unless we use our bodies, they literally waste away in a manner that resembles premature aging. Muscles deteriorate and grow slack; bones become more porous, brittle and easily damaged; the circulatory system loses its vigor and cannot cope with stress. After an accident, it is imperative to get back on your feet quickly to avoid compounding the injury with aftereffects.

In case after case, I have seen confirmation that after an accident, injury, or orthopedic trauma, acupuncture dramatically speeds recovery. By all means, when an emergency occurs, seek conventional medical attention, but do not stop there. Get your injured body to an acupuncturist as soon as possible.

REFERENCES

Two books that will tell you more about acupuncture and orthopedic trauma are Feng Tian-You's *Treatment of Soft Tissue Injury with Traditional Chinese and Western Medicine* (1983) and Bob Flaws' *Hit Medicine* (1983).

Chapter 9

INTERNAL MEDICINE

Over the centuries, Traditional Chinese Medicine has evolved into a system of theory and practice for treating all the ills and injuries that the body is prey to. It is based on experience, careful experimentation, trial and error, and observation. Unlike Western medical doctors, the acupuncturist treats every patient as a unique constellation of balanced energies; diagnosis and treatment of each case is tailored to the individual. Nowhere is this philosophy better illustrated than in the treatment of those disorders that Western Medicine labels "internal medicine."

Metabolic problems such as diabetes do not confine themselves to digestion but extend to almost all the other body systems as well. Acupuncture in the treatment of diabetes improves circulation, adjusts hormone production, regulates appetite, decreases urinary flow, reduces blood pressure, and restores general vitality. Changes brought about by acupuncture can help to minimize or eliminate the need for insulin in some cases.

Pat was middle-aged, overweight, and diagnosed with diabetes and hypertension. She had resolved to lose weight to improve these conditions, and she had heard that acupuncture might help. Like so many other overweight Americans, she had tried a series of useless diet regimens.

After examining Pat in my office, I concluded that her circulation was a big problem, no matter what other ailments she had. Circulatory imbalance appeared to be the underlying cause of the dark color and leathery texture of the skin on her legs. Poor circulation, she said, had bothered her for many years; she had difficulty walking and had pain in her feet. She had told her doctor that she was worried about her legs, but he had assured her that her circulation was adequate.

We began a series of treatments by needling points specified for this particular configuration of symptoms. Her skin softened and went from darkest red-purple to white. The hard, shiny surface and pitting owing to fluid accumulation disappeared—and so did her foot pain. She could walk normally. But we still had her metabolism to work on. When we began treatment, Pat's glucose levels were elevated, as were her blood pressure readings. With regular treatments over the next several months, we charted her blood pressure as it steadily dropped. Every four weeks, blood serum readings were checked, and they too dropped. As her general state of health returned, she not only began to lose weight, but she also experienced beneficial "side effects." Her opthalmologist reported a more normal pressure behind her eyes.

Studies of problems like this have shown acupuncture to be remarkably effective. In a Chinese study, acupuncture was used to treat twenty-three diabetics suffering from diabetic peripheral neuropathy. Patient's symptoms and signs of peripheral nerve degeneration improved significantly. Acupuncture treatment was so successful in all cases that for the first time researchers began to consider diabetic neuropathy to be a reversible condition.[1]

Similarly, in an American study, acupuncture was administered to thirteen hypoglycemic (low blood sugar) patients who were experiencing fatigue, headache, coldness, vertigo, tremors, and depression. Some progress had been made by following special diets that excluded sugars and were high in protein and low in carbohydrates and liquids. But needling treatment from one to thirty weeks relieved symptoms for all patients. Eleven patients were able to resume eating regular foods without discomfort, and their glucose tolerance tests were normal.[2]

Rita was plagued by lung problems for many of her 68 years. Weakened by chronic bronchitis, her lungs were susceptible to one infection after another. She never seemed to fully recover; she had a chronic cough and had difficulty bringing up the phlegm that clogged her throat. When she did so, it was an unhealthy color, often tinged with blood.

Complicating her condition were sinus headaches, sensitivity to cold, damp, and wind, and a low energy level. Western medicine might consider these symptoms unrelated, but not so in Chinese medicine. Appropriate treatments in Rita's case took somewhat longer than usual because her condition had persisted for seventeen years before she came to me. Still, she experienced a measurable reduction in her symptoms. Her chronic cough was gone and along with it her fatigue. Now when a bronchitis attack occurs, she comes for one or two brief treatments and recovers.

Joan sought help for asthma. In her 40s, she had just been released from a hospital where she had been given large quantities of cortisone for her breathing difficulty. On her first visit to me, she brought along her breathing machine, her oxygen, and her drugs. Frightened of leaving her house and taxing her lungs, she dared not make the short trip without her equipment. She was ready to try acupuncture because all else had failed.

Her progress in the next three weeks was remarkable. She no longer required oxygen or the breathing machine. She discontinued expensive drugs and nasal sprays. In a short time, she could venture out of her home, without paraphernalia, to enjoy her former activities. In the following three weeks, she was back to work, breathing easily.

Allergies, such as those suffered Ken, a labor organizer, also respond to acupuncture. In the summer and fall, he always suffered from familiar complaints: itchy eyes, sneezing, running nose, difficulty breathing, and insomnia. He came to me for a half-dozen treatments and experienced his first truly enjoyable summer in years, We have worked together now for three seasons, and he has booster sessions at the end of each winter, right before the spring allergy season.

Studies from around the world confirm acupuncture's effectiveness in treating respiratory problems. A study from Poland followed a group of sixty-four patients with chronic bronchitis. The program consisted of a series of once-a-week acupuncture treatments alternating with two or three months of no treatments. All patients had taken corticosteroids for a period of two to twenty-four years. Of the thirty-six who completed the three-year study, 64 percent were able to dispense with steroids and breathe normally.[3]

Nearly one-fifth of all the problems internists encounter are digestive disorders. These disorders take many forms, from simple inflammations through cancer (which I discuss in Chapter 10). Most problems in the digestive tract resolve quite well with needling.

Mary had a sixteen-year history of colitis, with characteristic symptoms of loose stools. She took four different medicines every day to control the colitis. When she was under stress, the medications did not help. Once we began treatments, we also began slowly weaning her off drugs. It worked. She had normal stools regardless of whether her day had been stressful. With needling, she has managed to discontinue 80 percent of the medications and feels like a new person.

Kevin, on the other hand, had experienced a lifetime of disabling constipation. He was skeptical about acupuncture but was ready to try almost anything for relief. The prompt results needling provided astonished him. Until then, he had a bowel movement every ten or eleven days; now he had a regular pattern of bowel movement every other day. Chronic constipation like Kevin's has received some attention in acupuncture research. A Greek study reports that after just one treatment 65 percent of 175 patients were cured, and an additional 30 percent recovered after three to five treatments.[4]

Healthy kidneys purify more than a ton of water each day, eliminate toxins, and precisely adjust electrolyte balances (ionized salts such as potassium in body fluids). Centuries ago, Chinese doctors devised needling methods to remove toxins from the body and improve the body's resistance to those that remain.

Tim's was a case of borderline chronic kidney dysfunction. As a child, he had a long attack of rheumatic fever that kept him in bed many months. Now, at 45, he had ascites (severe abdominal edema) and decreased urinary output. He experienced constant thirst, a cold feeling in the lower half of his body, and also complained of low sex drive. He had a needling session once a week for five months, which is not an unusual length of time for someone whose condition had persisted so many years. Tim lost all the excess fluid—and 40 pounds! He no longer felt chilled, and his overall level of energy and well-being returned, as did his sex drive.

Ruth suffered from cystitis (inflammation of the bladder). She had become thoroughly demoralized from bouts of discomfort, hospitalizations, and catherization. Still in her early 20s, she had nearly resigned herself to a lifetime of suffering. After only a few treatments, she had pain-free urination. Two years later, her freedom from symptoms continues. She no longer requires drugs or catheters.

The acupuncturist knows that no two patients have the same constellation of symptoms and must not be treated alike. Treatment of hypertension illustrates how individualized a diseased state can be.

Theresa's was an especially debilitating case. Her blood pressure was not stable, even with the use of several medications such as a blood thinner, a diuretic, and a beta-blocker. Her blood pressure fluctuated between abnormally high and low levels. She complained of being unable to function for days at a time because of constant dizziness. During her first visit to my office she had to press her hands against the walls to steady herself as she walked. Seated, she had to change body positions carefully to keep from losing consciousness. We decided that treating the disabling dizziness had top priority. She had her first treatment, and I helped her to a taxi. She called the next day to report that when she had arrived home she was exhausted and lay down for a nap. Two hours later, she awoke with a clear head and no dizziness.

Over the next few days, the dizziness did not return. Theresa's self-confidence returned so strongly that she ventured off to Maine for a fishing trip with her family. She returned ready to resume treatments to regulate her blood pressure and reduce her dependence on drugs.

Sally's was a somewhat different case: the 25-year-old woman's high blood pressure had developed recently and abruptly. She had a family history of hypertension; several relations suffered from stroke, toxemia during pregnancy, and general ill health. She didn't want to face a lifetime of drug dependency and risk the long-term side effects of kidney and liver damage. The acupuncture she received was therefore of a preventive nature; it lowered her blood pressure readings and restored her peace of mind.

Some hypertensive patients experience very few or no symptoms, yet show consistently high blood pressure readings. This was true of Lois. At 55, she was on a regular course of diuretic and blood pressure medications. Because she had attacks of gout as a side effect, she was eager to try acupuncture to lower the amounts of medicine she had to take. Within six sessions, her blood pressure had begun to decline. With the help of her hypertension specialist, she triumphantly halved her drug intake. We continued treatment and monitored her blood pressure readings. Her drug dosage was within the acceptable range. Now Lois's blood pressure is regulated with a quarter of the medication she used to take, and she has had no attacks of gout.

A few more cases of varied sort illustrate the wide variety of "internal" illnesses I have treated. Bill had been a patient once before for stress and fatigue and now sought help with a new problem. Several

months before he called for an appointment, he began experiencing
dizziness, nausea, dull frontal headaches, and pressure in his head and
behind his eyes. He began a long series of tests and procedures in a process
of elimination. Sinusitis, brain tumor, ear infection, hypertension, or any
other likely ailments were all ruled out. He was eventually diagnosed with
a form of Menière's disease (recurrent and progressive vertigo).

Bill described in detail the vertigo or dizziness attacks, their
beginning and duration. Certain there was a good chance that acupuncture
could cure his disease, I laid out a course of treatment. With three months
of once-a-week needling and daily herbal medicines, the Menière's
disease completely disappeared.

A young student, Nora, who had attended a workshop I gave,
consulted me for a rather unusual condition. She suffered from severe
dryness; she had no moisture in her eyes or her skin, no perspiration, no
menstrual periods. Several specialists had been treating various aspects of
her overall body state. She took drops for the eyes, creams for the skin, and
medication for the gynecological problem. But all her symptoms were
worsening. She could not get a good night's sleep because she had to keep
getting up to put drops in her eyes. She grew worried and depressed about
her fragile health. I explained to her that all of these seemingly separate
problems were part of a total body energy imbalance and that acupuncture
could turn it around. She agreed to try. After one treatment, her eyes teared
again. After two more treatments she was perspiring again, and by the time
we had done six needling sessions, her menstrual cycle returned.

Skin problems can be a source of great anguish and discomfort. We
believe that skin disorders mirror conditions of the internal organ and the
blood. The focus in treatment is to cleanse the blood, improve circulation,
detoxify the system, and promote tissue regeneration. Working from the
inside out, change is gradual and permanent. Acupuncture can eliminate
the need for drugs, ointments, medicinal cosmetics and patent medicines.
I once treated a young man with a nine-year history of eczema, who saw
his skin clear up completely in eight treatments. He has had no relapse in
the last three years. In another case, a middle-aged woman who had
suffered facial acne all her adult life regained a healthy, clear complexion
with acupuncture treatments and herbal medicine.

The effects of acupuncture are not the same from person to person.
Since each of us is unique, this is no surprise. There is no way to predict
how you as an individual will respond to treatment. You cannot directly
compare yourself to others to predict what your exact response will be.

The specific number and location of points that receive needling and the diagnosis that prescribes them are geared to your unique biological balance. A certain amount of patience is required as well. Many of my patients notice changes soon after a small number of sessions, but the full effect of acupuncture is achieved at different rates for different people. Acupuncture will work for most of the complaints usually listed under "internal medicine." This is so whether the symptoms are severe or mild, recent or long-standing.

NOTES

1. Bi Xiaoli, Zhou Guolin, Wang Zuo, et al. "Therapeutic Effect of TCM on Diabetic Peripheral Neuropathy." *Chinese Journal of Integrated Traditional and Western Medicine.* 8 (2):84-86, 1988.
2. C. S. Chen. "Acupuncture Treatment of Hypoglycemia." *International Conference of World Medicine*, New York, March 19-28, 1982. Meeting Paper.
3. J. Sliwinski. "Patients Suffering from Chronic Spastic Bronchitis Treated with Acupuncture and Their Granulocyte Migration." *International Medical Acupuncture Conference*, London, May 4-8, 1986. Meeting Paper.
4. P. J. Kotileas. "Constipation and Acupuncture." *International Medical Acupuncture Conference*, London, May 4-8, 1986. Meeting Paper.

REFERENCES

To learn more, you could start with I. Veith's *The Yellow Emperor's Classic of Internal Medicine* (1972). Also informative is *Essentials of Contemporary Chinese Acupuncturist's Clinical Experiences*, edited by Y. Chen and D. Liangyue (1989).

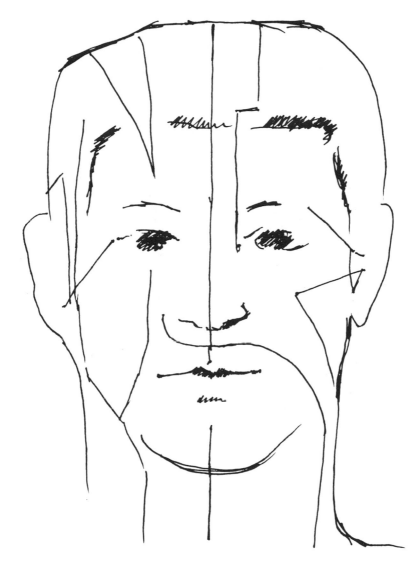

Some typical acupuncture channels on the human face and head.

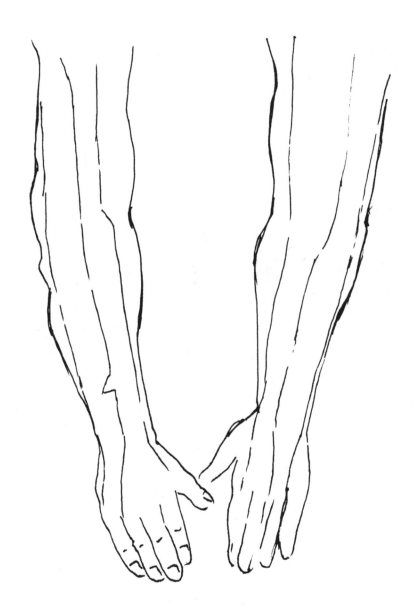

Some typical acupuncture channels on the human arms and hands.

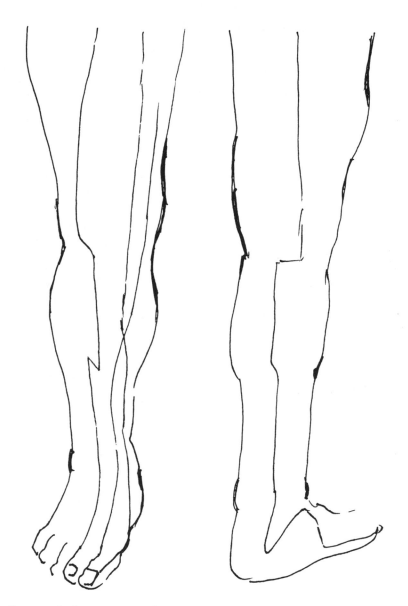

Some typical acupuncture channels on the human legs and feet.

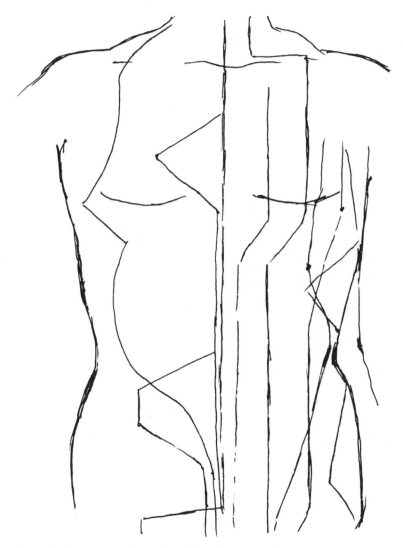

Some typical acupuncture channels on the human torso.

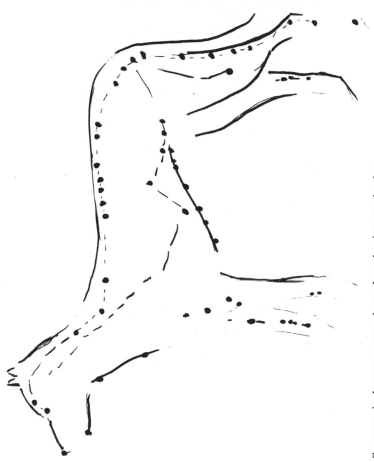

Some typical acupuncture channels and points on the dog.

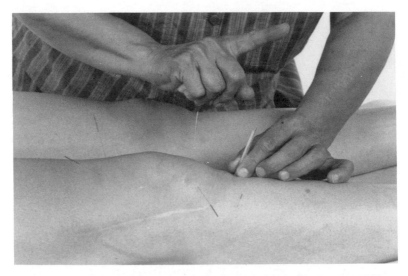

Needling by inserting through tube. Photograph © Martha Stewart 1993.

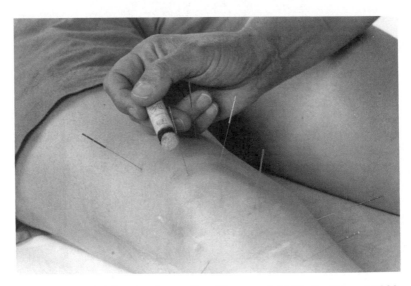

Herbal Moxa stick heating the needles. Photograph © Martha Stewart 1993.

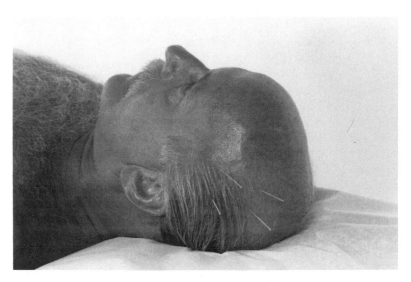

Needles in place for scalp acupuncture. Photograph © Martha Stewart 1993.

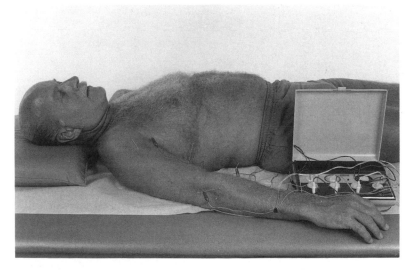

Electro-acupuncture. Photograph © Martha Stewart 1993.

Chapter 10

CANCER

Western medicine's treatment plan for cancer consists of surgery, chemotherapy, and radiation. Together, they have proven value but are not without grave side effects. Chemical agents used in treating cancer dangerously suppress the patient's immune system. Although the immediate effect of chemotherapy on some tumors is beneficial, the long-term consequences can be debilitating, even devastating.

Over the last decade, doctors treating cancer patients in China have developed a more benign strategy. They combine traditional acupuncture, herbal medicine, exercise, and diet with conventional Western practices. In tandem, the two traditions work together to treat each patient as a whole, integrated being and produce a much brighter picture for the patient's future.

Western medicine objectifies reality by describing and measuring living beings according to a narrow set of physically observable properties. If Western medicine cannot measure a disease by some tangible, quantifiable test, it often presumes there is no disease. Western-trained doctors do possess workable remedies, but they are not very effective in treating generalized and comprehensive maladies. This is especially true when disease states are vague and share the symptoms of a number of distinct, presumably unrelated diseases.

Traditional Chinese Medicine starts from an entirely different concept of reality. At its core is a view of body energies. Experienced practitioners, using the subtle techniques in which they have been trained, can assess the status of a patient's total energy flow. Over the centuries, Traditional Chinese Medicine has learned to tap into these energy resources in order to restore their balances. The body then has the opportunity to heal and reconstruct itself.

We practitioners do not deny or dismiss the effects of material reality—parasites, viruses, bacterias. Nor do we stop there: we add our own energetic levels of reality. The combination of the two medical systems has been more effective than either treatment working alone. Nowhere is this more apparent than in the treatment of cancer.

Both medical traditions agree that cancer is the abnormal multiplication of diseased cells. This perspective, however, deals only with the surface of the disease. We in Traditional Chinese Medicine continue looking for the "root" of cancer's cause in a predisposition to cancer. The root of cancer lies in the body's inability to maintain its natural balance. Cancer is a condition in which the pathology is out of control. As it progresses, the speed and intensity of its course may require immediate attention. Surgery, chemotherapy, and radiation are the tools for treating urgent, life-threatening symptoms. Traditional Chinese Medicine, including acupuncture and herbal medicine, takes effect more gradually and cumulatively. It brings about changes at a very deep, energetic level. But these changes require more time than a patient in acute, immediate crisis can spare. So, Western medical techniques may help to put an abrupt end to the disease process, and acupuncture and herbal medicine can support the person before, during, and after conventional treatment.

Whenever acupuncture and herbs are added to surgery, drugs, and radiation, Chinese doctors have found that prognosis can improve by up to 50 percent. How is this possible? Traditional Chinese Medicine treats cancer by (1) enhancing the working of conventional medicine (such as drugs and radiation) in the elimination of tumors, (2) ameliorating the side effects of these conventional techniques, and (3) supporting the person throughout the treatment process and restoring health after it.

Traditional Chinese Medicine, in conjunction with Western techniques, attacks cancerous growths directly. Herbs and acupuncture further act to lessen adverse side effects brought about by conventional radical surgery, radiation, and chemotherapy: epigastric distention, nausea, vomiting, loose stools, phlegm retention, and loss of appetite. Other complaints relieved are shortness of breath, fatigue, oral ulceration, depression, insomnia, ringing in the ears, indigestion, dry mouth, and pain. Cancer patients usually experience a decreased number of leukocytes (white blood cells) and a decreased count of platelets (cells that adhere to each other to stem the loss of blood). Cystitis (bladder inflammation) may occur, as may dermatitis and hair loss. A suppressed immune system leaves patients susceptible to secondary infections. Other complaints are forgetfulness, weakness of limbs, and headaches.

The side effects of conventional treatment vary from individual to individual. Clusters of side effects may appear in any combination after therapy. Ideally, the patient should begin acupuncture and take herbs several days before conventional treatment starts and continue it throughout. While conventional medicine is destroying deadly tumors, Chinese medicine is strengthening the body to protect it against other pathogens. It is also defending other, uninvolved areas of the body susceptible to injury from the toxicity of radiation and chemotherapy.

In the treatment of cancer, release from debilitating side effects is particularly important because it frees the patient's energies to fight his disease. In a Chinese study of malignant cancer, acupuncture proved to be a good inhibitor of problems such as anemia and low white blood cell counts. Because patients ate and slept better, their recoveries were facilitated.[1]

Acupuncture and herbs have a long-tested history as an approach to cancer. As early as the twelfth century, classic Chinese medical texts included special instructions on treating swellings, ulcers, and necroses (the death of areas of tissue or bone). Medical knowledge was sophisticated enough to classify tumors with some precision: glandular, mobile, or stationary masses, warts and moles, myomas, localized and diffused masses, and distention resulting from masses. There were also detailed writings on what to observe in the patient afflicted with cancer. The patient may have lost his skin luster, may show changes in skin color and texture, and may have significant blockage between throat and stomach causing regurgitation of food. He may have phlegm, retention of fluid, pain, hiccups, wheezing, bloody cough, and a feeling of suffocation. Of course, each of these symptoms can occur in many diseases other than cancer, but it is the overall picture that leads to the diagnosis.

In Chinese theoretical texts, the causes ascribed to tumors are numerous and include an inherited predisposition to long-term organ changes, prolonged emotional disequilibrium, indulgences in alcohol, and an excessively fatty diet. Bacteria and viruses can be added to the list of causes; any one of these causes has the effect of throwing the person's energy system out of harmony.

Not only does acupuncture play a vital role in treating cancer, but it also seems to work in detecting its early presence. Drs. Hiroshi Motoyama and Tsumeo Kobayashi in Japan has been studying early diagnosis of cancer using acupuncture meridians. First, they screen for abnormal occurrences of tumor markers in blood serum, which show up as changed patterns in specific, known enzymes. The earlier the cancer diagnosis, the more effective the treatment.

Dr. Motoyama began to investigate acupuncture meridians and points and compare them to their blood serum/biopsy methods. They chose specific points on the ends and beginnings of meridians and monitored these points with a thermal device.

They applied heat to twelve points, and subjects reported when they began to feel warm. The time required to feel heat in a healthy person is fairly uniform, about fifteen seconds. A longer lapse, say twenty-five seconds or more, at any one point on one or both sides of the body indicates that an abnormality exists. If a checkpoint showed such response, the researchers suspected disharmony, perhaps cancer.

Checking outpatients diagnosed with cancer by conventional techniques, the Japanese scientists measured their meridians for pathological signs. The standard biochemical and acupuncture assessments were in accord in a high proportion of cases. Thus, a person who displayed early signs of cancer also revealed abnormal readings on the acupuncture points. Acupuncturists then went on to treat these patients with vitamins and herbal medicines, and used special balancing techniques along acupuncture meridians. Of course, we do not know if further cancer growth was prevented in this way, but further follow-up of these patients may reveal some answers.

Once cancer has been diagnosed, Traditional Chinese Medicine can have an important role to play in its treatment. Larry, a 50-year-old man, had symptoms of nausea and experienced pain around the liver region; he had been unable to taste his food for over a year. Liver function tests showed abnormal readings; doctors suspected he had chronic hepatitis and treated him accordingly. His condition did not improve, and eventually masses were detected. Further testing revealed an enlarged liver with cancerous tissue. Because the area of the lesion was large, chemotherapy was begun. When Larry's blood showed a sharp drop in white blood count, the treatment was considered too risky to be continued. He then chose to try acupuncture and herbal therapies. At the beginning of treatment, he complained of severe abdominal distention, vomiting, dizziness, general lassitude, and difficulty walking.

For the next two years, Larry took his treatments and selected herbal medicines, and his condition gradually improved. His blood tests returned to normal levels. Stabilized, he continued treatment to improve his appetite and regain body weight. The area of pathological mass became smaller. Larry was able to return to half-time workdays. After eight years of treatment, he tests normal and appears healthy.

Peter, diagnosed with esophageal cancer, was administered a course of chemotherapy. When doctors found the cancer spreading to the sternum and chest area, they acknowledged that chemotherapy was unsuccessful and discontinued it. Because of difficulty breathing, Peter's doctors contemplated surgery, just to correct this respiratory problem. However, he was so weakened and his health so unstable that surgery was postponed.

Peter was also anemic. He could not sleep. He could not eat solids, and even a liquid diet disagreed with him. When drugs for this condition proved difficult for him to take, he sought acupuncture to relieve his pain. During six months of needling therapy, he began to eat normally and regained 40 pounds. Not only had his red blood count returned to normal, but his breathing problems and insomnia had disappeared as well. Furthermore, an esophagoscope exam showed regression of tumors. After another month of acupuncture, Peter was discharged and returned to work. After four years of periodic acupuncture and checkups, his tumors are still in regression.

Jules sought medical advice because of intolerable abdominal pain, blood in his feces, malaise, and general emaciation. Pathology samples and X-ray examination confirmed a diagnosis of rectal cancer. Radical surgery was performed and supported the initial diagnosis of a poor prognosis. After his discharge from the hospital, Jules's general condition was poor. He looked sick, and he continued to experience abdominal pain, distention and stomach discomfort, anal prolapse, loose stools, and poor appetite. His doctors, however, believed that the cancer was in remission.

Two months after surgery, Jules began a program of acupuncture and herbal medicine. He had some intermittent chemotherapy, and over the next five years he steadily regained his health. With continuing

Traditional Chinese Medical treatment, the other symptoms faded. He began to eat regularly, so that his body weight was restored and his vitality recovered. His resistance to everyday illnesses improved. Regular and recent checkups reveal no signs of relapse or spreading. Altogether, it has been fourteen years since the original, devastating diagnosis, and Jules's life remains on course.

Finally, Frank's history illustrates the value of acupuncture as a long-term means of maintaining health, once it is regained. When Frank developed a high fever and severe cough, his doctors hospitalized him for pneumonia. His was a stubborn case. Showing no improvement for two months, Frank was rediagnosed as having lung cancer. At the same time that he began herbal and acupuncture treatment, the entire right lobe of his lung was surgically removed. A month's course of radiotherapy followed. His regimen of herbal medicine and needling continued, enabling him to eat properly and allowing his body to recover from both the cancer and the radiation. That experience is several years behind him now. Frank continues regular periodic acupuncture sessions and takes herbal medicines to stay healthy.

Traditional Chinese Medicine can play an indispensable role in the treatment of cancer. Long-term cooperation between acupuncturist, physician, and patient improves the odds of beating the cancer. The patient can contribute a willingness to take responsibility in his diet, his activity levels, and his mental attitude. When symptoms show signs of disappearance, the patient should realize that a program of maintenance must be continued. Acupuncture will mobilize the body's curative capacity during and for a long time after illness.

NOTE

1. Xia Yuging et al. "Reaction Due to Radiotherapy of Patients with Malignant Tumor Treated by Acupuncture." *Chinese Acupuncture and Moxibustion.* 4 (6):6-8, 1984.

REFERENCES

The most up-to-date sourcebook is Dai-Zhao Zhang, *The Treatment of Cancer by Integrated Chinese-Western Medicine* (1989).

Chapter 11

THE IMMUNE SYSTEM AND ACUPUNCTURE

Acupuncture is wonderfully equipped to regulate the immune system—the body's defense against invasions. Let's look at modern research data on acupuncture and immunology and some practical applications. Because immunology is an enormously complex subject, I will provide details on only a few specific problems that I've encountered in my practice, among them rheumatoid arthritis, multiple sclerosis, and AIDS.

In a general way, your immune system has the capacity to discriminate between your body and agents entering your body that do not "belong" there. The defense process takes place in many locales: in blood cells, cell fluids, and circulating cell bodies. Defense activities also take place in digestive and respiratory tissues, as well as in bone marrow, saliva, and even tears. All of these areas play a role in keeping body processes healthy. Nonspecific processes destroy and devour pathogens such as viruses and bacteria. These defense agents are found in blood, lymph nodes, liver cells, the peritoneum (the lining of the abdominal cavity), the spleen, and body fluids—which are among the most important sites.

Normally, our bodies battle foreign pathogens and protect against something going wrong. We have the resources to fight a cold as well as tumors. Our bodies routinely handle such invasions. When we remember that the human mouth and saliva contain countless bacteria and other harmful agents that never succeed in causing damage, we realize how successfully this ongoing defense system operates.

However, a deficiency in the immune system can erode defenses, producing a number of unfortunate changes. Hypersensitivity or an abnormal reaction to a pathogen can develop; allergies are familiar examples. Autoimmune disease is another example in which the body develops antibodies against its own tissues. Immune defects allow pathogens to enter the body so that infections occur. An immune deficiency can allow the development of malignant cells within the body, which multiply unchecked. On the whole, Pasteur was correct when he speculated that the pathogen is peripheral and that the terrain (body environment) is central to disease or health. Potentially harmful agents will cause no damage as long as the place in the body where they intrude is doing its job in destroying or expelling them.

Finally, our immune system is affected by emotional states. Grief, bereavement, and stress can reduce response and raise the risk of disease.

For many years, both laboratory and clinical research has documented the effects of acupuncture on the immune system. Certain points can be needled to increase the "helper" T blood cells. Acupuncture also has a positive influence on patients' peripheral blood lymphocytes, substances that are important in the production of circulating antibodies that help to promote immunity against foreign bodies. Leukocyte (white blood cell) counts and mobility through the body have been found to increase by 168 percent within three hours after treatment. These "scavengers" help combat infection. The bactericidal power of plasma increases after needling. Acupuncture increases the number of cells that ingest and destroy bacteria, protozoa, and cell debris. IgM is an antibody found in blood serum that is effective against invading microorganisms. IgM cells quadruple over the days following treatment.

For centuries, Chinese doctors studied and wrote about febrile diseases. Their theories gradually evolved into a discipline all of its own. Wu You-ko, in the seventeenth century, specialized in epidemic diseases and classified them into febrile diseases and epidemic febrile diseases (noninfectious and infectious). He concluded that all openings on the surface of the body provide an entrance for communicable pathogens. Yeh

Tien-shih, in the late eighteenth century, built on this work and developed treatments for feverish diseases. In the same century, Wu Tang concentrated on diagnosis of diseases; he divided diseases according to the pathological symptoms and signs each displayed. In the nineteenth century, Lei Feng classified feverish diseases into seasonal pathogens and designated appropriate treatments. Chinese doctors also described the depth and severity of illnesses and developed treatments for all levels of febrile diseases.

Chinese practitioners spoke of "guards" in fighting feverish diseases. These guards exist as a form of surface energy. Quick and mobile, they respond to and repel invasion by outside agents. Practitioners also developed the concept of the "army camp," which they thought of as powerful repositories of energy, slower to mobilize but always ready to take on any large-scale invasions. These immune functioning aspects, still called *Wei* and *Ying* energies, respectively, depend in turn on reservoirs of energy located in body organs and fluids. The main goal of both the doctor and the patient was to keep the Wei and Ying robust and in balance. To accomplish this objective, doctors prescribed proper diet, exercise, rest, and moderation of passions. They also administered herbs, applied needles, and burned moxa.

Ancient Chinese ideas about superficial and deep immunities are relevant today. The immune system is constantly being called upon to deal with viruses, bacteria, and various pathogens, and most of the time it eliminates them successfully. But if the invasion enters a chronic phase, it engages the immune system in a different way. Then the internal organs are severely weakened and the prognosis for recovery greatly reduced. The modern Western approach has been to use drugs—chemical sledgehammers. It is common to use dangerous steroids and repeated rounds of antibiotics and combinations of drugs. Such drastic therapy is given to already weakened patients; scant attention is paid to strengthening and revitalizing the patient. Diseases that are an expression of an altered immune response may be more effectively treated by acupuncture and herbal medicine. A large number of clinical and experimental studies have proven that numerous complications that result from weakened immune response or that follow surgery can be controlled and completely cured with acupuncture. Acupuncture has been used to successfully treat the following conditions:

Cellulitis   Infection in or close to the skin which spreads through

	the connective tissue
Erysipelas	Localized inflammation and redness of the skin and underlying tissue
Lymphangitis	Inflammation of lymph vessels, frequently caused by streptococci
Thromboangiitis	Inflammation of a blood vessel with clot formation
Folliculitis	Inflammation of follicles such as hair on the scalp or face
Lymphadenitis	Inflammation of the lymph nodes due to buildup of toxic substances

When used postoperatively and as prevention or treatment for infection, needling is an effective anti-inflammatory measure for all of these conditions.

Another area in which acupuncture has been profitably used is in the management of acute gastroduodenal ulcer. Acupuncture is applied as the main method in the acute stage to relieve serious pain, enhance body resistance, and promote healing of the perforated intestinal wall.

Acupuncture has been used to counteract many kinds of poisoning. It has been effectively used in treating radioactive research accidents, drug poisoning, and anaphylactic reactions such as poisoning by antimony (a metal used in alloys and some medicines), and penicillin anaphylaxis (severe allergic reaction). Needling can help in treating carbon monoxide poisoning, chronic benzene poisoning, and poisoning from agricultural chemicals, nitrates, and spoiled foods.

In addition to these assaults on the immune system, there are also categories of patients who are vulnerable to infections. Individuals with acquired immunodeficiency syndrome (AIDS) are greatly at risk. The AIDS virus destroys many aspects of the immune system, and as a result the body becomes weak and is easily infected. Cancer patients are also especially susceptible to infections due to an underactive immune system. Malnutrition and radiation treatment weaken the immune system. In addition, cancer cells produce chemicals that may limit the ability of the body to defend itself. AIDS and cancer patients easily develop such immune system breakdowns as herpes zoster and fungal infections. Patients who undergo organ transplants are at risk of infection owing to the very drugs that are used to prevent rejection of the transplanted tissue/ organ. These drugs also suppress the growth of vital defense cells. Diabetes patients have weakened immunity resulting from abnormal glucose metabolism. Finally, kidney disease prevents adequate filtering of toxins of all types. All of these conditions and susceptibilities are helped by acupuncture.

Acupuncture, either alone or in combination with conventional treatment, can slow down and even reverse degenerative diseases. Multiple sclerosis (MS), rheumatic disease, and lupus have all been studied in regard to any benefits needling could provide. A study from the former Yugoslavia reported satisfactory results in twenty-eight patients ranging in age from 24 to 60 years. An American study of arthritis concluded that it seems evident that acupuncture, with little or no side effects or complications, should be considered as an alternative treatment for arthritis because of its pain-alleviating effects and suppression of inflammation.[1,2]

Lupus is another disease that responds to acupuncture. In a survey of international studies done on lupus patients, favorable results were reported on rheumatic disease symptoms and the boosting of the immune system. Patients also managed stress better, showed less fatigue, and ran fewer risks from the side effects of steroid medications.[3]

In my practice I have treated both animals and humans with autoimmune diseases. One case was a young woman with MS. At the point she sought my help, she was experiencing pain and loss of mobility in all four limbs. At the end of ten treatment sessions, one per week, she had no pain and had regained mobility and energy.

The success of acupuncture on rheumatoid arthritis has depended on the length of time the disease was entrenched in the body. One case I helped was that of a woman in her mid-40s, diagnosed with the disease ten years before. She was European and told me that she traveled throughout the continent in search of release from her pain. She finally discovered acupuncture. Treatments provided the pain relief she needed to live comfortably and care for her family. Her weekly sessions had kept stiffness, joint swelling, pain, and deformity at acceptably low levels. Now that she was in the United States for a prolonged stay, all of her symptoms had returned. We agreed on several treatments scheduled very close together to deal with her immediate discomfort, followed by a weekly management plan. She began to feel better after the first session and continued to improve rapidly. We continued sessions for three months until she returned home to her regular practitioner.

AIDS is one of the most devastating forms of an immune system disease. It has rapidly assumed epidemic proportions, capturing attention in the news media and promoting radical changes in our social behavior.

Although AIDS is caused principally by the infection of a pathogen, accompanying factors determine the speed of deterioration of the immune system. Among these factors are constitution, diet, stress, and substance abuse. After becoming infected, people with AIDS have erratic health histories; they dramatically move back and forth between periods of relative well-being and bouts of numerous opportunistic infections. Treatment is available for most of the specific infections, but nothing is yet effective against the AIDS process itself. As a result, many AIDS patients are seeking alternative treatment methods.

Several Chinese medicine clinics have begun work with AIDS patients in the large metropolitan areas of New York, Boston, Chicago, and San Francisco. Nearly all of their patients have used other treatment modalities by the time they receive acupuncture and herbs: experimental therapeutic drugs, nutritional programs, and exercise. The therapeutic protocols and goals in the clinics are, first, to produce an antiviral effect as a result of strengthening the immune system, and then to modify the external and internal factors that may affect the course of the disease. Each AIDS patient is considered a unique individual. Each receives a special diagnosis rooted in the specific needs of his body energies. Treatment is then tailored to the patient's requirements.

Statistics collected over the last ten years demonstrate that Chinese medicine has achieved dramatic and reproducible benefits for AIDS patients. Among these are mitigation of fatigue, improved breathing and sinus drainage, diminished size of lymph nodes, and diminished or eradicated night sweats, diarrhea, pain, nausea, and skin irritations. Acupuncture has reduced the pain of Kaposi's sarcoma, a kind of malignant growth seen in the late stages of the disease. Chemotherapy patients report fewer side effects when they coordinate their chemotherapy with needling. Acupuncture also addresses another serious AIDS-related problem: emotional distress marked by depression, anger, and fear.

Perhaps the most beneficial result of acupuncture is prophylaxis management. Most practitioners believe that it is important to use acupuncture to enhance the overall health and vitality of those at high risk of developing AIDS. We also believe that it is essential for patients with early diagnosis of HIV or AIDS to enter long-term, Traditional Chinese Medicine programs in order to improve and prolong their quality of life. Two cases of AIDS patients illustrate the success of the process.

Wes had developed herpes zoster. His pain was severe enough to keep him from work. One treatment brought the pain under control; a second session prevented new lesions from forming and cleared up existing ones. He returned to work within a week, after having been on sick leave for three weeks.

In another patient, Stan, the virus attacked the optic nerve. He had lost the vision in his right eye about a year before coming to me. Even with the use of new, expensive experimental drugs, Stan was rapidly losing the sight in his left eye, too. A course of acupuncture twice a week and herbs taken daily began to slow the rate of vision loss. Within three weeks after the first session, Stan's eye stabilized. For the next four months we continued regular therapy and he maintained his level of vision. Unfortunately, he contracted pneumonia. He was hospitalized for two weeks and then moved into hospice care, so that he was no longer able to receive acupuncture treatment. A month after needling was discontinued, he became blind.

I have discussed some of the more serious diseases that Chinese medicine has been able to help. In my practice, I have found that acupuncture and herbal medicine are the only cure for the common cold and viral flu infections. If used at the very earliest signs of these common ailments, or used preventatively after exposure to pathogens but before symptoms appear, acupuncture and herbs work 99 percent of the time to abort the attack. After a flu or cold begins, either acupuncture or herbs can shorten the length of illness. In more severe cases, when a cold or flu lingers, producing a heavy cough, sinus infection, and fever, acupuncture still helps. It can alleviate an ailment that has become deeply entrenched in the body.

If you suffer every winter with bronchitis, chest problems, or asthma, or if you experience allergies each spring, then a short series of treatments just before the season will elevate your immune system and may prevent recurring ailments. One of my patients, Dennis, had originally come to me for a knee problem. He decided to try a preventive plan, and for the last three winters he has not had to endure his "yearly" bout of bronchitis.

Martha first came to me for treatment of her headaches. She decided to do something for her allergies. Before her allergies began, she had a series of six treatments to desensitize her system; she needed no medication that spring—nor the next one, nor the next.

Peter, a ten-year-old boy, had a flu that quickly developed into Bell's Palsy, which caused left-sided facial paralysis. His doctor told him that he would be fine, or at least better, in a few months. Meanwhile, the little boy could not blink, control tears from the left eye, or even eat normally. I gave him five treatments and within two weeks his face was back to normal, and he was thrilled that he could whistle again.

In more virulent, acute infections, Chinese medicine can lessen both the intensity and duration of the symptoms. For example, a diabetic patient of mine who was receiving treatment for that condition developed a painfully infected toe. She began treatment with antibiotics but experienced no improvement. After just two acupuncture sessions and with an herbal ointment and herbal soaks, the toe returned to normal.

Bladder infections or cystitis are terribly painful, so that sufferers need quick relief. Most dash off to the doctor for a course of antibiotics. Sometimes this works, but often it backfires. The cystitis recurs repeatedly, so that more and more antibiotics are needed to cure it. Acupuncture, on the other hand, has a very good record for treating acute and chronic cystitis. When used in conjunction with diet supplements and herbal remedies, the infection disappears rapidly.

I also treat people who have chronic viral infections for which Western medicine has afforded no relief. I have successfully treated Epstein-Barr virus, mononucleosis, and chronic fatigue syndrome (CFS), all of which are debilitating and take unrelenting hold of the patients' systems. One such case was that of a young woman with CFS who had been to several clinics in the area, had received a variety of drugs, and had even joined a support groups for CFS sufferers. She had read up on alternative treatment and badgered her doctor into making a referral. He referred her to me. I gave her a short series of four needling sessions and worked out a long-term program of herbal remedies and supplements. Over the next three months she was encouraged enough by her improvement to continue therapy. In just three more months she was well enough to accomplish two goals she had postponed: she went back to work full time, and she got married.

What is the role of Chinese medicine in treating immunological disorders and infections? In life-threatening situations, I do not hesitate to recommend conventional therapeutic drugs such as antibiotics. These drugs can effectively deal with immediate life-or-death situations. But practitioners of Chinese medicine utilize needle points and herbal prescriptions that can treat serious infections and fevers and can be used in conjunction with antibiotics. Acupuncture helps in cases of meningitis, encephalitis, endocarditis, rheumatic fever, malaria, pericarditis, nephritis, and syphilis.

Chinese medicine not only attacks specific diseases, but it also helps promote the general health of the patient, thereby helping increase his or her strength to fight disease. The same is true for diseases where conventional therapy has had a poor record of success. Diseases such as MS, lupus, myasthenia gravis, arthritis, and chronic immune deficiency appear to be caused by imbalances of body energies. This lack of underlying harmony appears to Western medicine merely as a mysterious and vague set of symptoms with no easily isolated cause or agent. For these illnesses, a subtle diagnosis made by an experienced practitioner can indicate treatment that helps body parts work together to counter the disease. Acupuncture stimulates multiple interdependent body systems to start repair work. It changes labels like "obdurate," chronic," and "intractable" into "healed."

NOTES

1. A. Steinberger. "Specific Irritability of Acupuncture Points as an Early Symptom of Multiple Sclerosis." *American Journal of Acupuncture.* 14 (3-4):175-178, 1986.
2. M.H.M. Lee, Gai-Fu Wm. Yang. "The Possible Usefulness of Acupuncture in Rheumatic Disease." *Clinical Rheumatology in Practice.* 3 (6):237-147, 1985.
3. Feng Shu-Fang, et al. "Treatment of Systemic Lupus Erythematosus by Acupuncture." *Chinese Medical Journal.* 98 (3):171-176, 1985.

REFERENCES

For a thorough review of Traditional Chinese Medical knowledge about immunology see Dr. Hong-Yen Hsu and Su-Yen Wang, *The Theory of Febrile Diseases and Its Clinical Applications* (1982).

Chapter 12

GYNECOLOGY AND OBSTETRICS

Traditional Chinese Medicine (TCM) sees the human body as the product of an orchestral performance in which all the parts work together to produce a balanced, harmonious concert. This is the natural state of affairs for the human body. No one instrument—body part or function—dominates, plays out of turn or rhythm, or plays too loudly or softly. Disease in the body is akin to a state of disharmony in which one instrument or section insists on upsetting the equilibrium of the whole, disrupting the entire performance. The practitioner of TCM is analagous to a conductor who restores balance so that all the instruments play their proper parts in the prescribed way.

TCM practitioners restore balance by considering each individual's state of health as unique. No two persons are alike, even though on the surface they many seem to suffer similar symptoms or illnesses. These symptoms may conceal differences in underlying imbalance, and for this reason each patient must receive individualized treatment. Acupuncture has little in common with the assembly-line care offered in most conventional clinics, doctor's offices, and hospitals.

Finally, TCM has always recognized what physicians in the West are only now beginning to acknowledge—prevention is the highest form of medicine. By visiting their acupuncturist when they anticipate that some medical problem may arise, people in China take full advantage of the preventive side of acupuncture. In the West, however, most patients rarely seek out an acupuncturist until some problem has developed and generally after they have failed to get relief by conventional means. It is wise to use acupuncture as a regular part of your health care rather than wait until desperation drives you to seek help.

Women are special cases, with menstruation, fertility, pregnancy, birthing, and menopause all exclusively features of female bodies. (Fertility can be a male issue also.) When any of these features is not as it should be, a woman feels the dysfunction is a disease of her entire body. She is in pain, food has no taste or makes her nauseous, she perspires excessively, she has diarrhea or constipation. She feels vaguely angry, resentful and ill-tempered. In short, she feels thoroughly miserable. TCM views gynecological disharmony as an impairment of the flow of Energy and Blood. Neither is being distributed throughout the body in its proper volume. The flow is depleted or excessive, or the amounts are excessively clustered in inappropriate locations. Only when the circulation of Blood and Energy is normalized will the woman's body function harmoniously again and her symptoms be dispelled.

A painful menstrual cycle will usually respond to acupuncture therapy. Dysmenorrhea, or painful menstruation, has many forms, but pain is the common ingredient. It can occur in the abdomen, back, legs, or head. In some women, it is coupled with severe fatigue and depression. Menstrual periods can be painful in as many ways as there are women. Chances are good that acupuncture can relieve them all, not only alleviating present pain but also ensuring that future periods will be pain free.

One patient who came to me had been diagnosed as suffering from endometriosis (abnormal sites of lining tissue in the pelvis or abdomen). She had experienced occasional discomfort when she first began menstruating, and as the years passed this escalated into daily, continuous torment. She said, "I had pain every day. I had gone the drug route, which left me worse off, plus having terrible side effects. I was on the pill, and it gave me headaches." The hormone treatments her gynecologist prescribed left her nauseated, constipated, and exhausted. She decided to try acupuncture as a final measure. She had avoided it because of her fear of needles, but this was easily overcome. During the course of six treatments, her symptoms began to disappear; nausea and constipation ended, digestion improved, and her headaches stopped. Soon it was possible to dispense with the hormones and regulate her period by acupuncture alone. Her pain has not returned; her cycle is normal. The breast tenderness and backache are just memories.

Menstrual pain need not be endured as "normal." Two separate studies done in England and Italy compared groups of women who received acupuncture with control groups who did not. Those treated with needling showed a 90 percent rate of improvement over those who were not.[1, 2]

Amenorrhea, the absence of a menstrual cycle, can be long-standing or recent. One of my patients, a woman in her early 30s, had not had a period in ten years. She had been examined by many gynecologists, none of whom had been able to do more than prescribe drugs, which she was reluctant to take. After eighteen treatments over a twelve-week course, she began menstruating regularly and predictably. A year later, she phoned to report that her cycle continued to be normal and painless.

Another patient developed amenorrhea after a long history of irregular periods. Her gynecologist told her that she could never conceive because of it. Only after a friend urged her to see me did she consider acupuncture. The first goal was to restore her period, which was accomplished after about ten treatments. We then began a second series of sessions to regulate her cycle. During these treatments, the intense cramps she experienced at the onset of menstruation disappeared. Her course of treatment lasted three months, with one treatment each week. For the first time in years she felt like a normal woman—and within two months of her last treatment she became pregnant.

Premenstrual syndrome (PMS) is an affliction that occupies a curious niche in Western medicine. There is no straightforward test for it, and it cannot be diagnosed solely by its symptoms, all of which occur with other ailments. Since PMS cannot be clearly isolated and defined, it is little wonder that Western medicine has no effective treatment for it. Nowadays one sees frequent television ads for patient cures that make inflated claims to ease this mysterious disease. Often, the usual treatments—hormone medications, dietary changes, stress management, vitamin supplements—are either not able to combat the ravages of PMS or do so only temporarily. For millions of women, PMS breaks the month into two parts, one of which is beyond their control.

One of my patients, Cathy, lost physical coordination during PMS attacks. A week to ten days before her period, she would walk as if intoxicated. Her vision and motor abilities were so disrupted that she dared not use any tools, not even scissors. She would gain as much as five pounds, usually as fluid retention, so that her clothes did not fit properly. She slept badly. During ten weeks of treatments, her symptoms disappeared, one by one. She now comes to me for a preventative session every other month to sustain her healthy equilibrium.

Anne was another PMS victim. For half of every month her breasts were swollen and tender. She could not stop binging on sweets and junk food. Hers was an extreme, though not an uncommon, story. She related that PMS had driven her husband from her and was threatening her relationship with her boyfriend. She needed help desperately. For half a month she was happy, patient with her children, capable of working and enjoying life. Then, as if a switch were flipped, she would be irritable, screaming at everyone. All she wanted was to be left alone with a box of chocolates. Unable to cope with this split life, she took the advice of a friend who recommended acupuncture. After having a treatment a week for two cycles, everything changed. If she hadn't plotted herself on a calendar, she wouldn't have known she was going to have a period. The periods came and went with no exhaustion and no emotional roller coaster ride. Anne now returns to my office every few months for a brief treatment to maintain the health she has achieved.

For Anne and for others like her the endocrine system plays a key role in PMS. That is why Western doctors prescribe hormones. Acupuncture, on the other hand, deals with the hormonal influences of PMS by inserting needles at certain points of the body to restore equilibrium.

Western scientific evidence has established that acupuncture causes the release of pituitary chemicals. It influences the hypothalamus, thyroid, adrenal, and gonad glands. Needling also affects the pancreatic islets and the parathyroid glands. Controlled clinical and experimental evidence collected from around the world during the past thirty years supports the view that acupuncture stimulates and regulates all these glands so that they naturally and in combination produce hormones necessary to the balanced functioning of women's reproductive systems. Any woman who wishes to eliminate or prevent costly occurrences of PMS will benefit from simple and unobtrusive acupuncture.

Becoming pregnant, staying pregnant, staying well during pregnancy, and delivering a healthy baby without complications are all part of a well-functioning reproductive system. Chinese medicine encourages women to seek care before they conceive because it is so much easier to avert potential troubles in advance.

How can a woman know she is a candidate for a problem pregnancy? One indicator is a history of painful or irregular menstrual cycles. Obesity, anemia, or eating problems can contribute to child-bearing difficulties, as can generally poor health and a low energy level. A woman who has had a miscarriage can unquestionably profit from acupuncture in planing her next pregnancy.

During pregnancy, acupuncture can clear up any of the long list of problems that commonly appear: morning sickness, spotting, fluid retention, urinary problems, and pain. My colleagues and I treat depression, chronic cough and respiratory congestion, allergies, cystitis, and elevated blood pressure. Just about everything that can go wrong during a pregnancy may be effectively and simply corrected so that the pregnancy is comfortable.

Lynn found it extremely difficult to stop smoking during pregnancy, even though she felt she must. She tried hypnosis and nauseating drugs—all to no avail. Three needling sessions of about twenty minutes each broke her addiction. Another patient was in agony with severe allergies. Her physician's advice was to learn to live with the symptoms because the only drugs that might help her could also harm her unborn baby. A friend encouraged her to come to me. After her first session, the discomfort diminished dramatically; by the end of the third treatment, it was gone completely.

At the eighth month of Diane's first pregnancy, her hands became painfully swollen. The pain lasted all day and kept her awake at night. Medication was out of the question, and her obstetrician told her the condition was untreatable and just had to be endured. Some of her co-workers had been patients of mine and urged her to try acupuncture. Over the objections of a skeptical husband, she phoned me for an appointment. I began treating her, and she was back to normal after two treatments.

Carla, another patient, had experienced spotting from almost the beginning of her pregnancy. She was in her fourth month of pregnancy when I used needling and appropriate herbal medicine. After two treatments, she completed the rest of her term comfortably and gave birth to a healthy baby.

Breech presentation, difficult and prolonged labor, retention of the placenta, and hemorrhaging are all problems that can endanger either mother or child but can be corrected by acupuncture.

The method of reversing feet-first to head-first presentation is quite simple. The patient is treated daily for up to four days at a point on her small toes. Two energy channels that balance the internal and external energy flows of reproduction connect at these points. Blood tests of women who have been needled here show significant elevations of certain hormone levels. After needling, the fetal heart rate increases, and the frequency and range of fetal movement go up, reaching a peak within one to several hours after treatment. The baby spontaneously reverses itself at the peak of this activity. This treatment has had extraordinary success: one Chinese study of one thousand women reports that six hundred and seventy-three cases were corrected with acupuncture—a success rate of 67 percent.[3]

Acupuncture is not helpful in some very rare cases—for example, if there are uterine deformities, or if the baby's head is fixed in a position beneath the mother's ribs. Apart from such rare circumstances, however, acupuncture is a safe and risk-free alternative to expensive hospital stays and surgery for breech presentation.

Rupturing the membranes surgically to induce labor carries with it the risk of infection. Labor-inducing drugs can have harmful side effects for the baby. Electro-acupuncture runs no risk to mother or child and has no harmful side effects. When obstetricians use drugs to start labor, their success rate is about 70 percent; acupuncture achieves a 72 to 80 percent success. An entire course of labor can be maintained without complications or artificial means. Most women need no painkillers throughout the first stage of labor and only very low levels of analgesia toward the end. The vital signs remain normal, and the average induction and delivery time lasts about thirteen hours.[4]

Acupuncture anesthesia was first used in China for Caesarean sections in 1966 and has now become quite common for such deliveries. Unlike conventional drug use, it is free of complications and side effects. Chinese doctors favor it for patients whose pregnancies are complicated by hypertension, toxemia, and convulsions because acupuncture anesthesia stabilizes blood pressure, lessens blood loss during surgery, and has none of the risks of conventional chemical anesthesia. Recovery after surgery is quick. Women use smaller amounts of painkillers after the incision and suffer less from gas distention. Results are more satisfactory when the section is anticipated and planned, when it is the mother's first delivery, and when surgery lasts no more than thirty minutes. Acupuncture allows the woman to be fully conscious and alert throughout the birth so that she can participate in the entire experience painlessly.[5]

Acupuncture is seldom considered a cure for infertility, although it is a remarkably effective treatment for it. Acupuncture stimulates the production of glandular chemicals in the hypothalamus; this in turn activates the pituitary gland, which produces both follicle-simulating hormone (FSH) and leutenizing hormone (LH). In the female, FSH is necessary in the development of fertile eggs and of estrogen. LH continues the work of maturing the eggs and manufacturing progesterone. The two hormones work together to regulate normal cyclic changes in the female reproductive system. In this way, ovulation is promoted and regulated, and pregnancy is possible.

In males, FSH and LH increase fertility by producing mature sperm. LH helps develop testosterone, the hormone essential to the development of a mature male. Acupuncture treatments significantly raise the concentration, volume, and motility of sperm. Research studies provide statistical evidence for increased fertility in both males and females through acupuncture. In one report of twenty-four functionally sterile women, eighteen began ovulating after acupuncture and sixteen became pregnant. Another study reports that eleven males in a group of thirty-two showed improved quality of sperm.[6, 7]

Hormone production and ovulation decline in the years preceding and following menopause. These changes can continue for an extended period of time. Coupled with other factors such as general health, quality of diet, level of activity, and genetic makeup, they can produce a wide range of symptoms, some of which are severe or disabling. Acupuncture can bring relief to women suffering form hot flashes, insomnia, fatigue, or low sex drive. Nan came to see me when she became alarmed by changes taking place in her body. She was in her late 40s, and her once regular cycle was skipping months. She perspired heavily day and night regardless of weather. After a half dozen treatments lasting a month, Nan returned to menstruating regularly for an entire year with no further distressing symptoms.

Traditional Chinese Medicine can solve most of the problems women encounter from puberty to menopause, and it does so without risk, a factor that is especially critical during pregnancy. One study assessing the role of therapeutic drugs taken during pregnancy found that mothers who had taken synthetic hormones, tranquilizers, or antibiotics during pregnancy were 50 percent more likely than nonusers to have malformed babies. Acupuncture could easily have been substituted for any of these drugs. Similarly, medical news continues to question the advisability of hormone treatment for women during menopause because of ill effects and the yet-to-be-determined long-range risks of hormones.[8]

Acupuncture is effective in treating many other gynecological ailments. For example, chronic inflammatory pelvic disease has a cure rate of about 60 to 88 percent.[9] In research on fibrocystic breast disease, an average of eight needling sessions has been shown to be enough to dissolve cysts in nearly 95 percent of cases treated.[10]

Sandra's history is complex and helps illustrate many of the subjects I have touched on here and in other chapters. Because every individual is unique, her experience did not fit neatly into a single compartmentalized category. Sandra's mother referred her to me. Sandra and her husband had been trying to conceive for several years without success. After a program of eighteen weekly treatments, she missed a menstrual cycle. She had a positive pregnancy test and called me with the happy news.

My advice was to combine my care with that of her ob/gyn practitioner. I believed this cooperation to be especially important in her case because Sandra entered the pregnancy as a high-risk patient. She weighed nearly 280 pounds; she was hypertensive, and she had an enlarged heart and chronic nephritis. I drew up a plan of weekly treatments and herbal remedies for the first trimester. Her ob/gyn monitored her blood pressure and other signs every week at a local hospital.

Sandra completed the first trimester with no problems; she experienced no rise in blood pressure or kidney problems; and she had no physical discomfort or fatigue. I recommended that we drop down to an every-other-week needling schedule, and I altered her herbal prescriptions for the second trimester. For the third trimester, we changed the strategy again to anticipate and prevent problems such as toxemia. We returned to weekly acupuncture sessions and added some new herbs.

Sandra sailed through with absolutely no problems. She had a comfortable full-term pregnancy and even worked at her job up to the last week. She delivered a healthy baby boy.

NOTES

1. J. M. Helms. "Acupuncture for the Management of Primary Dysmenorrhea." *Obstetrics and Gynecology.* 69 (1): 51-56, 1987.
2. N. Bondi, R. Albo. "Dysmenorrhea Treatment with Acupuncture of 40 Cases Personally Observed." *Minerva Medica-Minerva*

Riflessoterapeutica. 72 (33):2227-2230, 1981.

3. Fu Jing-Chang, et al. "Clinical Observation of 1000 Cases of Pregnant Women with Breech Position of Fetus Treated by He-Ne Laser Radiating Zhiyin Point." *Chinese Acupunture and Moxibustion*. 7 (5):1-2, 1987.

4. E. Yagudin et al. "Acupuncture During Childbirth: Fetal and Maternal Effects." *International Medical Acupuncture Conference*, London, May 4-8, 1986. Meeting Paper.

5. Acupuncture Anesthesia Group. "Caesarean Section Under Acupuncture Anesthesia." *Chinese Acupuncture and Moxibustion*. (5):13-15, 1983.

6. Yu Jin, Zheng Huaimei, Ping Shengmin. "Changes in Serum FSH, LH and Ovarian Follicular Growth During Electroacupuncture for Induction of Ovulation." *Chinese Journal of Integrated Traditional and Western Medicine*. 9 (4):199-202, 1989.

7. Zhang Jiasheng. "Male Infertility Treated with Acupuncture and Moxibustion: A Report of 248 Cases." *Chinese Acupuncture and Moxibustion*. 7 (1):3-4, 1987.

8. G. Greenberg, W.H.W. Inman, J.A.C. Weatherhall, A.M. Adelstein, and J.C. Haskey. "Maternal Drug Histories and Congenital Abnormalities." *British Medical Journal*, Oct.:853-6, 1977.

9. Wang Xiaoma. "On the Therapeutic Efficacy of Electric Acupuncture with Moxibustion in 95 Cases of Chronic Pelvic Infectious Disease (PID)." *Journal of Traditional Chinese Medicine*. 9 (1):21-24, 1989.

10. G. S. Chen. "Acupuncture Treatment of Breast Fibrocystic Disease." *International Conference on World Medicine*, New York, March 19-28, 1982. Meeting Paper.

REFERENCES

Two books by Bob Flaws about acupuncture and gynecology can enrich your knowledge: *Free and Easy: Traditional Chinese Gynecology for American Women* (1986), and *Paths of Pregnancy* (1983). For detailed information on classic and modern approaches, see *A Handbook of Traditional Chinese Gynecology* (1987), compiled by the Zhejiang College of Traditional Chinese Medicine.

Chapter 13

PEDIATRIC MEDICINE

Diagnosis of children is difficult, because little patients cannot describe their symptoms as accurately and in as much detail as adults. To make a diagnosis, then, the practitioner must rely on looking, feeling, pulse-taking, and asking the subject and parents about the condition. Parents are often distressed and may not be able to provide helpful on-the-spot information. Thus, much of the required information comes from nonverbal sources. Children are easy to treat, however, because their illnesses are usually simple, and they heal quickly.

We practitioners of acupuncture start by checking the patient's face and eyes, facial color, body movement, and skin quality. In children, these areas can change rapidly and are reliable indicators of health. We look at the mouth, tongue, ears, eyes, and nose, and ask parents about the anal and urethral orifices. We are looking for such indicators as discharges, inflammations, skin changes, and color. For example, dark circles around the eyes point to specific channel problems.

We examine the inside edge of the index finger, where the child's entire pulse system is located. This technique dates back at least 1,500 years. The pulse helps provide information on the depth of the invasion of a disease and suggests a prognosis. By feeling the skin at several locations, we judge the temperature. We also listen to the child's voice and breathing. The questions we ask of parents concern elimination, digestion, sleep, and pre- and postnatal health history.

In Traditional Chinese Medicine, pediatrics deals with a varied repertoire of ailments. A great many childhood ailments involve digestion or a spleen disharmony. Indicators of this problem are vomiting, diarrhea, constipation, poor appetite, and tiredness. In addition, children may be more susceptible to respiratory problems; these can include asthma, ear infections, and sinusitis.

Children are by nature more active than adults and thus function more at the yang pole of energy harmonics. Accordingly, they are less affected by cold and cold diseases, and they are more prone to fevers and convulsions. Children are delicate, however, and are easily affected by environmental factors: overheating, changes in diet, catching chill. Childhood illnesses also progress quickly. There is a maxim in our medicine that says, "easily ill, easily cured." Fortunately, although children's illnesses can progress rapidly, they respond quickly to treatment. This axiom is also applicable to emotional problems. It is easy for a child to fly into a rage and make herself sick. Children are also sensitive to the emotional states of those around them. Severe emotional trauma or prolonged emotional excess will upset channel energies, which in turn can disrupt organ systems.

Of course, there is a broad range of congenital abnormality that is not due to any trauma, but these, too, can be helped with acupuncture.

Acupuncture, particularly in the West, is not widely used in the treatment of children. This is a pity, because TCM can effectively cure a great many childhood ailments. There are many misconceptions about pediatric acupuncture. Laypeople, and some pediatricians, too, imagine that acupuncture hurts babies and young children, but they are mistaken. Acupuncture is a benign procedure. Used with skill and caution, needles are relatively painless, and therapy can be started a few days after birth. Acupuncture has a more pronounced curative effect on children than on adults, so that less therapy is required. Children are more yang, with greater energy flows, and that gives needling a more profound and lasting effect.

Acupuncture can be used for both acute and chronic syndromes and for common disorders as well as rare afflictions. Americans are usually surprised at the list of illnesses that acupuncture can help. Needling is appropriate for common childhood ailments such as mumps, tonsillitis, conjunctivitis, earache, and measles. Needling can help sleep disorders such as night terrors and bedwetting and is effective with respiratory sicknesses such as bronchitis, pneumonia, childhood asthma, influenza, and coughs. Endocrine disorders such as pancreatitis, childhood diabetes, and abnormal growth patterns respond well. The same is true for neurological problems such as convulsions, epilepsy, mental retardation, and paralysis. Children respond well to treatment of dermatological problems such as eczema and dermatitis. Numerous studies on these and more serious illnesses show astonishing improvement with the techniques of TCM.

In a Chinese study of infantile diarrhea, 1,102 babies were treated once a day at two points for three days. All of these patients had been previously given antibiotics and fluid infusions with no success. With acupuncture, the cure was complete in 86 percent of the subjects.[1]

In another report, fifty-two German children suffering acute sinusitis were divided into two groups. One group was treated with acupuncture, and the other group received conventional therapy of inhalations, antibiotics, or vasoconstringent nose drops. The report concluded that far more effective results were achieved by acupuncture.[2]

A Chinese study was done on thirty-five children with hydrocephalus, or accumulation of fluid in the head. Most of them had a history of vomiting and diarrhea, and a few had convulsions. Other symptoms included enlarged head circumference, bulging fontanelles (the large cranial plates at the top of the head), distended scalp veins, and a splitting of cranial sutures (the natural closings of the bones). In addition to a disproportionate head-to-face ratio, the children had muscular weakness, and impaired vision, and a few showed mental retardation. Skull X-rays showed evidence of chronic increase of intracranial pressure. All of the children received acupuncture with the number of treatments ranging from 10 to 240. The results, 84 percent effective, were measured by echoencephalograms and X-rays.[3]

Another Chinese study concentrated on retarded children, treating five hundred and fifty-eight cases. All patients were treated for four months. In the beginning twenty days, the needling was performed once daily, and after that, once every other day. The effect was evaluated after four months. There were one hundred and twenty-seven cases with marked effect, three hundred and fourteen with improvement. The lower the age and the longer the treatment course, the better the effect.[4]

Although vaccines have nearly eradicated infantile paralysis in this country, a Chinese study reports on one hundred and one children treated for the sequelae of this dread disease. Nineteen were completely cured. Marked improvement took place in fifty-nine children, and partial improvement in another twenty-two. Acupuncture was ineffective in only 1 percent of cases.[5]

A Russian study of school children with slight to severe myopia (nearsightedness) demonstrated that acupuncture had stopped the progress of myopia, normalized the condition and improved vision acuity.[6]

One interesting study addresses the problem of deaf-mutism. One hundred and twenty-five cases were treated with needling once daily. A minimum of twenty-six and a maximum of seventy-eight sessions resulted in twenty-seven cases being cured, seventy-nine cases improved.[7]

In Canada, Dr. Mario Wexu has started a free clinic for congenitally deaf children. Under the supervision of the Institute for the Deaf and Dumb, acupuncturists treat children once a week. Results are measured by the children's regular physicians as well as the Institute doctors. Some of Dr. Wexu's patients have had up to 40 percent hearing improvement after six months of treatment. The average rate of improvement for all cases, after ten treatments, is 15 percent. Very few cases failed to respond at all. Dr. Wexu believes that if treatment could be administered more often each week, as in China, recovery would be faster. There, where the recovery rate is 80 to 90 percent, treatments are given every day for ten days, with a three-day rest period before resumption. The longer the treatments are received, the greater the success. Dr. Wexu himself uses only two points per treatment, alternating local points around the ear with points away from it, on the arm or hand.

A 1991 acupuncture study of cerebral palsy followed sixty-five children aged from forty days to seven years. All of the children were hospitalized in the first year of life and from their examination results were diagnosed with cerebral palsy. In this study all forms of cerebral palsy were represented: spastic, dyskinetic (slow, involuntary movement of the extremities), hypotonic (weakness in coordination, unsteadiness) and mixed. Some children had problems in all limbs, some predominantly in the legs or arms. Needling was performed on body and scalp points. Both electro-acupuncture and laser acupuncture were used. Treatment was directed to head control, extremities, hypersalivation, speech abnormalities, and strabismus (optic nerve problem).[8]

Treatment was arranged either daily or two to three times a week, depending on individual severity. Treatment lasted four months with management therapy for up to five years after initial results. During the five years of observation the researchers reported the following results: in sixty-one cases (94 percent) considerable improvement was observed, and in four cases (6 percent), complete recovery.

An ongoing program in Hungary at the Akupunkture-Rehabilitation Foundation in Budapest, and in former Czechoslovakia at the Prague Teaching Hospital, Department of Physiotherapy, has developed out of a study of babies damaged by oxygen deprivation (hypoxia). In 1991 Drs. M. Lidicka and G. Hegyi (of Hungary and Czechoslovakia, respectively) reported on a two-year study of their treatment of one hundred and forty-five handicapped children suffering from hypoxia. Like their Chinese colleagues, the doctors found that early treatment improved chances of success. Dr. Hegyi began treatment ten days after delivery and found that babies who were treated under the age of a year- and -a-half did not require institutionalized care. Babies in this program are treated three to four times weekly, and some do not even need physical therapy. In newborns, acupuncture serves to support the infant's life and prevents spasms and other disorders. Closest attention is given to the limbs and back, but the face is also needled to stop grimacing. Once the child begins to show improvement, the frequency of needling is reduced.

A final report concerns an ongoing American project in Santa Cruz, California: the PRES (Physical Response Educational System) program directed by Jeanne St. John, Ph.D., through the county Office of Education. The project has two main goals: to use acupressure on handicapped children and to train therapists, teachers, and parents in the use of this technique. (Acupressure is hand stimulation of points.)

The children in this project are severely to profoundly developmentally disabled, emotionally disturbed, and orthopedically handicapped. Many suffer from cerebral palsy, Down's syndrome, birth defects, and other neurological disorders. A pilot study was begun in 1980, in which a group of patients were treated with acupressure massage. Within six to eight sessions, some changes were noticeable: 74 percent of the children improved in all four diagnostic areas: sensory/motor, cognitive, social/ emotional, and general health.

Dr. St. John writes, "One 9-year-old with CP (cerebral palsy) crawled, sat, stood, walked, and spoke for the first time. One 13-year-old learned to play soccer, swim, ride a skateboard, use gym bars, all for the first time. Another 13-year-old improved 2 to 5 grade levels in math and language, and went from 40 percent to zero absence rate. A 17-year-old went from echolalic speech to simple sentences. A 9-year-old went from temper tantrums daily to none."[9]

In the diagnostic categories, the following improvements were recorded:

1. Sensory/motor: There was improved muscle relaxation and control, and there were fewer involuntary movements. Children developed finer motor control and better hand-to-eye coordination, and could better follow rhythm, balance themselves, and write.
2. Cognitive/communication: Students initiated language and increased their vocabularies, concentrated better, and were able to complete their homework. Their visual/auditory memories were improved, as were their speech and reading.
3. Social/emotional: General compliance and behavior were improved; children were more sociable and happy, less aggressive, and less frustrated. They had fewer tantrums and cried less, and their motivation improved.
4. General health: Less bedwetting, fewer allergies, and more infrequent asthma attacks were noted. Chronic pain was reduced; digestion improved along with bowel control; and self-injurious behavior ceased.

As teachers and administrators in the county school district and other California districts became aware of the PRES achievement, requests for information and for training in acupressure flooded in. Parents wanted to learn how to administer followup sessions themselves. Teachers of handicapped students wanted to employ the miraculous technique themselves. In response to these requests, Dr. St. John has begun giving workshops to parents, educators, and health care practitioners. One of her greatest success stories took place at the Pearl Buck School in Oregon. Starting with a small number of profoundly handicapped children, her trained assistant began using daily acupressure massage as part of the total education plan. Results were so satisfactory that now every child in the school has an acupressure session once a week. I might add that in China, acupressure is a routine part of nursery, kindergarten, and elementary school programs. Routine massage of their own eyes to improve vision is one part of such programs.

I have treated a number of hyperactive children. All had problems concentrating, learning, playing quietly alone, and getting along with siblings and playmates. Some had aggressive tendencies, and some had bedwetting problems. The behavior of some of these children worsened in reaction to certain foods, and many of them had sleep difficulties.

All of my hyperactive patients have been males under 8 years of age. All underwent a short series of needling treatments, to which none objected so strongly that we had to stop. All have showed a cessation or significant reduction in characteristically hyperactive behavior and in associated health problems. All have been mainstreamed in their schools. Several of my patients who had been in "special needs programs" were mainstreamed upon evaluation the year after treatments. Those who were about to enter school were allowed into regular class levels. A couple of my patients have gone on to become high achievers in school. They have done well in their course work and are self-motivated, nonaggressive, delightful children—and drug-free.

Enuresis (involuntary urination) is frequently encountered in children and it does not respond well to conventional methods of treatment such as drug therapy, psychotherapy, conditioning, or surgery. A study from Romania reported that in one hundred and eight children ranging in age from five to nineteen years, the results of needling treatment were 34 percent remission for over one year. In another 38 percent, the frequency of nocturnal involuntary urination decreased to less than once per week.[10]

Earlier in this chapter I discussed the positive results of acupuncture in treating hearing problems. A rewarding case of mine was a 10-year-old who was becoming progressively deaf. His pediatrician had advised waiting until his condition progressed to the point that he could be fitted with a hearing aid. Over the course of twelve treatments, my patient showed genuine improvement. He could hear better in the classroom, and he was able to hear whispers and discern very soft high and low tones. When he went for reevaluation, his physician was astonished by his improvement—both subjectively and as recorded on hearing tests. Now I see the boy four to five times a year to ensure his continuing progress; he has never had to endure the awkwardness of wearing a hearing aid.

Even in China, many children do not receive treatment until their disorders have become severe. These young patients have frequently not been helped by conventional remedies. Some patients have had severe afflictions since birth. Yet, even in these "worst case" problems, the effectiveness of acupuncture has been remarkable.

Chinese medicine is definitely effective in dealing with common childhood ailments: tonsillitis, mumps, and respiratory and digestive disorders. Acupuncture can also cure a wide range of "behavior" problems, from persistent bedwetting to disruptive hyperactivity. Finally, great benefit is to be gained by using Chinese medicine preventively, to ensure from birth onward, a happy, healthful childhood.

NOTES

1.   He Jingzhi. "Infantile Diarrhea Treated with New Acupuncture Therapy." *Chinese Acupuncture and Moxibustion*. 6 (93): 4-6, 1986.

2.   H. Eichner, G. Kampik, M. Wimmer. "Acupuncture in Acute Sinusitis Maxillaris in Children and Adults." *Akupunktur Theorie and Praxis*. 15 (1): 6-4, 1987.

3.   Chen Xuenan, et al. "TCM: Survey of the Effect of Acupuncture Therapy in Thirty-Five Cases of Obstructive and Communicating Hydrocephalus." *Journal of Traditional Chinese Medicine*. 7 (2): 101-104, 1987.

4.   Jin Rui, et al. "Observation on the Therapeutic Effect of 558 Cases of Hypophrenic (Retarded) Children Treated with Acupuncture in Sishen-Points (4-Mental Points) and Zhisan-Points (3-Intelligence Points)." *Chinese Acupuncture and Moxibustion*. 12 (2): 3-6, 1992.

5.   Ren Shouzong. "Acupuncture Treatment for Sequela of Poliomyelitis." *Chinese Acupuncture and Moxibustion*. 1 (1): 38-39, 1981.

6.   I. V. Valkova and O. Y. Nyurenberg. "Electroacupuncture in Myopia." *Vestn. Oftalmology*. 1 (33): 1989.

7.   Xhang Zhaoying. "Observations of 125 Cases of Deaf-Mutism Treated with Acupuncture." *Chinese Acupuncture and Moxibustion*. 10 (2): 6, 1990.

8.   Wojciech A. Filipowicz. "The Application of Modern Acupuncture Techniques and Methods on Children with Cerebral Palsy." *American Journal of Acupuncture*. 19 (1): 5-9, 1991.

9.   Jeanne St. John, "Acupressure Therapy in a School Environment for Handicapped Children." *American Journal of Acupuncture*. 15 (3): 228, 1987.

10. C. Ionescu-Tirgoviste, Visinescu Rodica, Ionescu Camelita, M. Tomescu. "The Treatment of Enuresis by Acupuncture." *American Journal of Acupuncture*. 11 (2): 119-124, 1983.

REFERENCES

The use of acupuncture to treat childhood ailments is discussed in detail in Bob Flaws's, *Turtle Tail and Other Tender Mercies: Traditional Chinese Pediatrics* (1985). See also J. Scott, *The Treatment of Children by Acupuncture* (1986). A comprehensive article by Dr. St. John, "Acupuncture Therapy in a School Environment," can be found in the *American Journal of Acupuncture*, vol. 15, No. 3, 1987.

Chapter 14

VETERINARY MEDICINE

Eddie is a giraffe. He lives in Windsor Safari Park just outside London, England. For about a year Eddie had suffered from arthritis and walked with a painful-looking limp. The humans involved in Eddie's life, the park director and head veterinarian, were unable to help much. The two men scheduled a trip to China, and there they observed acupuncture being performed on large domesticated animals. They paid particular attention to the work being done on arthritic cows. The veterinarian couldn't wait to return to try the techniques out on Eddie. After a few treatments on his leg, Eddie began to walk without a limp.

Large and small domesticated animals can be helped with acupuncture. These cures have a high rate of success, and they can be accomplished at significantly less expense than conventional veterinary surgery. If you have ever had a pet who required surgery or long-term health care, you know that the cost can be astronomical.

Consider the case of an older golden retriever who had been hit by a car. She sustained a hip fracture, shock, and paralysis. She was in severe and continuous pain. Initially, the veterinarian surgically repaired the hip and leg and administered antibiotics. The dog showed some improvement;

however, she could not bear any weight on the leg and foot, and lesions on the foot refused to heal. She was referred to me after the cast was removed, and we began therapy. After three sessions, the dog began supporting herself on her leg. She continued treatment, and her coordination continued to improve. She was taken for longer and longer walks, and soaks and ointment were given for the lesions. Her owner has continued home treatment, and the dog shows signs of recovering normal use of her leg. Needling has saved the lives of countless animals; truly, good medicine for humans is also good medicine for animals.

In the Paleolithic age, humans polished small, hard stones that they used to puncture the skin and draw out blood and infected tissue. Seeing that it worked on themselves, the next logical step was to apply this procedure to domesticated animals. In China, the first known veterinary medical texts date back 3,000 years and describe the use of acupuncture on elephants. With the development of Chinese bureaucracy, government employees assumed responsibility for the maintenance of animal health, and that of horses in particular. The father of this branch of medicine was Pao Lo, in the fifth century. Lo was the first full-time veterinary practitioner to use the new medicine based on channel theory, yin/yang concepts, and the 365 then-known acupuncture points.

By 220 A.D., there was a proliferation of medical writings on the care of cattle, pigs, camels, donkeys, geese, chickens, and, of course, horses. All of the major Chinese hospitals established schools of veterinary medicine. In the Sung Dynasty (960 to 1279 A.D.), the government opened the first "drugstores"—in this case, dispensaries of remedies—for veterinarians. Federally appointed officials had the responsibility of dispensing and controlling supplies. The growth of this thousand-year-old example of government-regulated medicine is easy to understand when we consider the economic value of livestock.

Two brothers, Yu Pen-Yuyan and Yu Pen-Heng, published their *Treatise on Horses* in 1606. The treatise is a record of their sixty years of practice, as well as a compendium of medical information from earlier times. The text has been the most widely circulated and most influential veterinary source for the last three hundred years in China. Its influence spread to Europe, and it was known to Claude Bourgelat, who included acupuncture in the curriculum when he founded university-level veterinary studies in France. Acupuncture was routinely practiced on small animals in Europe until the nineteenth century.

When swine diseases reached epidemic proportions in the Ch'ing

Dynasty (1644 to 1912), veterinarians soon developed comprehensive texts for treatment. These prescriptions and charts are still in use and are as effective today as they were three centuries ago.

With the formation of the Republic of China, Western-style veterinary medicine came into vogue. Even so, traditional medicine continued in rural areas. Then, with the Cultural Revolution in the 1950s, China encouraged a return to ancient medical techniques. The present government's policy was established by Chairman Mao Tse-Tung, when he stated, "...if the modern practitioners of human and veterinary medicine do not unite with the more than one thousand traditional practitioners and help them progress in knowledge and ability, they are in fact helping evil and letting humans and animals die of disease."[1]

Veterinary acupuncture was introduced to Korea in the sixth century and to Europe in the seventeenth century. Dr. E. Kampfer introduced acupuncture to Germany in 1683; Claude Bourgelat developed college-level veterinary acupuncture studies in Lyon, France. Acupuncture medicine had been introduced to France by Jesuit priests who served in Chinese courts in the seventeenth and eighteenth centuries. Interest in the medicine reawakened in the twentieth century when France became involved in Indochina.

The fiftieth emperor of Japan (who reigned from 482 to 507) sent an envoy to a Chinese university to study acupuncture, and the exchange continued to the present day. Since the 1950s, worldwide interest in animal acupuncture has markedly increased. In 1954 Dr. Masayashi Kirisawa, who runs a clinic in Japan, came to the United States to report on the care of horses. During his lectures, he reported that he treated fifty race horses a day with acupuncture.

Most treatment of humans applies to animals as well. Meridians and points are similar, and a wide variety of animal diseases and injuries can be treated with needling. There is one obvious difference: animals cannot talk about their subjective feelings and sensations, so the doctor must rely on observed external signs to judge the disorder and results. She must listen carefully for sounds of wheezing, stomach rumblings, teeth grinding, and other indications when making a diagnosis. The owner provides information on appetite, respiration, elimination, and signs of pain or discomfort. The doctor palpates (feels) various areas, points, and channels to gain information.

Treatment is simple and quick. Small animals are fairly easy to treat and usually lie quietly. Once the needles are in place and manipulated, the dog or cat enters a drowsy state and does not seem to mind the procedure. Needles can be heated or electrically charged. Large animals may require greater preparation such as physical restraint, but they, too, appear to tolerate the therapy well. Modern veterinarians have at their disposal electro-acupuncture for ailments such as paralysis. They also use laser acupuncture instead of needles and herbs instead of drugs. Acupuncture anesthesia is also employed for large and small animals.

Practitioners use acupuncture to treat reproductive disease, musculoskeletal problems, neurological, circulatory, and gastrointestinal disorders, and dermatological afflictions in animals. Acupuncture can work in cases where conventional medicine has failed or had to be abandoned because of great cost.

My first bird patient was Alice, a rose-breasted cockatoo. She was referred to me by her vet. She had a chronic bacterial infection in her gut that would not clear up, despite repeated series of antibiotics. Alice had lost her appetite, weight, and zest for living. Food passed quickly through her digestive tract, so she was becoming malnourished. Her owner was desperate and eager to try acupuncture.

Alice was a challenge to me. Aside from feeding wild birds, I had no experience with any birds and I knew only a little aviary anatomy. Furthermore, I had no acupuncture charts for birds. I realized that I would do no harm to Alice and that she was not going to survive without some kind of medical treatment that worked. In consultation with her vet, I decided on laser acupuncture. This would be fast and safe for such a fragile creature. Alice took her first session well; she did not fuss while being constrained, and after it was over in a few minutes, she showed no stress.

After six appointments, the content of her crop was examined for evidence of change, and all appeared normal. During the month I worked on her, Alice's health gradually improved. Her appetite returned, she gained weight, and by the end of her treatment series she was singing and flying about the house. She has remained healthy for the last three years. Until Alice's owner moved out of state, Alice came to me for a preventive program several times a year. Her endearing personality has raised my sensitivity toward birds in general.

Treating Alice gave me the experience and confidence to take on another cockatoo, a sulphur-crested fellow named Charlie. He had stopped eating, and his veterinarian had been force-feeding him for a week. I could see that Charlie was in pain by the way he held himself. Now that I was more certain about needle points, I treated Charlie aggressively just once on a Sunday morning. That night he was eating.

Most of my animal work is on larger animals, such as dogs and cats. Perhaps one of the reasons they are brought to me is that pet magazines often carry articles about the benefits of animal acupuncture. On the whole, the pets I treat respond well and quickly. They do not appear to mind needles, and following treatment they seem relaxed and mellow. When I lecture, give demonstrations, or write about animals, I stress the fact that acupuncture is a valid and viable alternative to conventional veterinary care. It can be used to treat virtually any ailment, not just hopeless situations or cases in which an animal is in severe pain.

Calvin was one of my first canine cases. He was a friendly labrador, prone to bloat, a serious problem that can kill a dog if not corrected. Because Calvin's bloating episodes had been so frequent, the owners were advised to have surgery performed. Based on reading they'd done, the owners opted for acupuncture. On our first meeting, they reported that Calvin had vomiting episodes and was very gassy. He seemed out of sorts, and was not his usual agreeable self. I did eight treatments on Calvin, at first a few days apart and then at longer intervals, while we monitored his progress. It has now been nearly six years since his first needling, and Calvin has not had a single episode of bloat. He never had the recommended surgery.

When I describe cases such as this in a lecture, pet owners listen in disbelief. Those who have had sick animals have been told that surgery is the only solution. I explain that, just as with humans, I work with the whole dog or cat, not just the isolated symptom. Owners can usually supply a long list of subtle and obvious ways in which their pet has changed, and these changes along with my examination help me form a diagnosis. My object is to alter the entire animal's chemistry so as to restore its body harmony.

Some cases are purely mechanical problems, such as with Fred, a corgi. Fred was paralyzed throughout his low back (lumbar) area and lower limbs. This had been his condition since he'd had back surgery. For several months afterward, his vet insisted that he would eventually walk again. Fred's owner took him swimming, lovingly massaged and gave physical therapy to his back legs, but the dog got no better.

After just a couple of acupuncture treatments, Fred began trying to stand on his hind legs. Two more sessions, and he could walk a little on one leg, dragging the other along. Following several more treatments, both legs began to work. The walking was ungainly, and Fred did stagger a bit, but we knew that communication between spinal cord and legs was returning. Gradually, Fred made a complete recovery. He was able to run and join in family play with his former gusto.

Relay, a Chesapeake Bay retriever, had a problem with vomiting. His owner believed that training for retrieving had made him a sick animal. For several years he regularly vomited both his food and bile. No dietary changes seemed to help. He had prolonged bouts of diarrhea, with mucous and blood in the stools. His disposition had changed too; he was not the affectionate, self-confident, happy dog he'd once been. His owner had taken him to a series of vets and clinics, with no improvement. Relay's owner had heard of me through breeders at a dog show and decided that acupuncture was worth a try. After an examination and diagnosis, we decided on a series of acupuncture treatments, supplemented with herbal medicines and dietary changes. The treatment plan worked, and Relay has recovered his health. If he gets off the track a bit, a dose of herbal medicine brings him back.

Acupuncture effectively treats pain in animals. Many dog breeds are prone to cervical degeneration and pain, hip dysplasia and pain, and painful arthritis. Willie the dachshund was a typical case. His veterinarian strongly advised surgery on his neck but admitted that the prognosis was poor. Because Willie's owners wished to spare him the discomfort of the operation and also because the proposed surgery was very expensive, they opted to try a few acupuncture treatments. They were amazed and delighted when Willie's pain completely disappeared. It has not recurred in four years.

It is not unusual when a cat refuses to eat occasionally, but Bear was one who gave it up altogether. He was given many kinds of tests, spent a week in the cat hospital, and came home with only a large bill to show for it. I gave him a single treatment in my office at about 5 p.m. one day, and later that evening he started to eat again. He was put on a single herbal remedy for a week's recuperation, and his eating problem never returned.

Animals can also suffer from uncomfortable and unsightly dermatological problems. A doberman named Edie had skin problems most of her life—a dry, itchy scalp, raised red bumps, and dandruff. Her owner had tried drugs and prescription shampoos with no relief. My comprehensive plan included a complete change in diet, a couple of acupuncture treatments, and herbal medicine. We watched and waited two weeks, during which time Edie's skin condition improved. Then I gave her one more treatment and more herbs to take. Now she is a new dog; people who do not know better mistake this glowing, healthy nine-year-old for a dog a third her age.

Related to these skin ailments is another condition that veterinarians usually find extremely difficult to cure: canine lick granuloma. Dogs will chew and chew at lesions on their body making them worse. I have treated dogs who have had cortisone therapy, surgery, implants, and even psychological therapy for this problem. Most of my canine patients heal well; three to six treatments, a topical herbal ointment, and herbal soaks seem to be all that is required.

Often I am asked to work on severe cases: liver or kidney failure, and cancer. My approach is to use an aggressive therapy of frequent treatments, together with herbs and natural remedies. One such case was Houlihan, a springer spaniel with a long history of seizures. He had been medicated with Dilantin, an antiseizure drug, which had begun to destroy his liver. His abdomen was full of fluid—a condition called ascites, which often accompanies liver failure. He was given about two months to live.

I gave Houlihan liver-regenerating herbs and put him on a vegetarian diet to give his liver a chance to rest. With his veterinarian's cooperation, Houlie was put on a different medication, at a lower dose, for the seizures. Then I needled him a couple of times a week for two weeks, afterward reducing this treatment to once a week. In the two months' time he had been given to live, Houlihan started to recover. All symptoms disappeared; the serum readings of his liver functions became normal. I continue to treat Houlihan occasionally with acupuncture and herbal medicines, both for his general health and his seizures. It has been five years since his first acupuncture treatment, and he enjoys an active 11-year-old's life.

One of the most gratifying aspects of veterinary acupuncture has been my work with older pets. The owners of these pets are always distressed by the animal's infirmities but understandably do not want to have them destroyed if possible. Sally, a 14-year-old mixed-breed dog, had a severe case of allergic dermatitis. She had lost almost all of her hair from her shoulders back to her tail, and she continually scratched and bit herself until wounds appeared that would not heal. All previous medical attention had had no effect. Sally was given fourteen treatments of electro-acupuncture, and over the course of the therapy the symptoms disappeared. Her skin cleared, and she sported a new coat of fur. She went on to enjoy a dignified old age.

I have described just a few cases of animal illnesses that I have helped in my practice using Traditional Chinese Medicine. The list could be lengthened. The whole gamut of ailments—some general and some specific to certain species and breeds of animals or birds—would fill the pages of a large book. Acupuncture and herbal medicine as practiced over thousands of years now constitute a body of knowledge and techniques capable of curing all manner of illnesses. All the principles that apply to treating humans work in veterinary practice. The care we practitioners can provide animals is comparatively inexpensive—an additional incentive to relieve helpless creatures of unnecessary suffering.

NOTE

1. Mao, T.T., 1953, 1032.

REFERENCES

To learn more about Traditional Chinese Medicine and animals, see S. Altman, *An Introduction to Acupuncture for Animals* (1981). Another good source is the book coauthored by A. M. Klide and S. H. Kung, *Veterinary Acupuncture* (1977).

For general information see T. T. Mao, *Quotations of Mao-Tse-Tung*, Peking's People's Press, vol. 3 (1953).

Chapter 15

OVERCOMING ADDICTIONS THROUGH ACUPUNCTURE

John had been a smoker most of his adult years. His experiences are typical of most people who use acupuncture to break addictions. He says, "I was a heavy smoker—about two and a half packs of cigarettes a day for thirty years. I didn't seem to have any of the obvious physical problems smoking causes except that I couldn't quit. I tried many times. The withdrawal symptoms, both physical and mental, were so intense that I finally gave up trying."

John's son gave him the present of an acupuncture treatment, hoping that it could accomplish what nothing else had. John came for the session early one morning and continued on his usual daily round. He recalls that "After 45 minutes driving to my office, I pulled into the parking lot and realized that I hadn't smoked in the car! I usually smoke a couple of cigarettes on the way to work.

"I started my day, and after three hours it struck me that I had not smoked once. There was nothing in my brain screaming for a cigarette. Now this was unusual. I was used to smoking a cigarette every fifteen to thirty minutes during my waking hours my whole grown life." John reported that he had no urge for a cigarette and that he awoke the next morning without an overpowering desire for a smoke. "I had already scheduled another acupuncture treatment close to the first," he remembers, "and believe me, I went. I haven't lit up since."

Addictions, whether to tobacco, alcohol, drugs, or certain foods, are tough to end. Conventional means for treating them are costly and often fail. There are smoking clinics that offer hypnosis or some variety of behavior modification. Some people choose to use "patches" that contain nicotine; others use doctor-prescribed nicotine chewing gum. The idea is to withdraw from nicotine slowly to ease the body's discomfort, a process called "tapering off."

Similarly, withdrawal from heroin or cocaine may be managed with methadone, but this substance is itself addictive, and the patient must be weaned away from it as well as from the primary addiction.

Overeaters have a smorgasbord of choices—weight loss programs, diets, medications, even surgery. All of these choices are expensive, and the results are usually short-lived. Can acupuncture help? Numerous reports confirm its success. In a Chinese study of four hundred and seventy-three cases of obesity, ear points were used with a 60 percent effect rate.[1] A Russian stop-smoking study reported 71 percent success.[2] An American study used acupuncture in place of methadone.[3]

In a slightly different U.S. study of patients who had become addicted to prescription painkillers, 85 percent withdrew from medication with no or minimal side effects after receiving acupuncture treatments.[4, 5]

How can an ancient medical technique successfully deal with modern epidemics? Why do a few slender needles inserted into the body or the external ear, and sometimes electrically charged, cause people to immediately stop drinking, drugging, smoking, or overeating? Frankly, no one understands the exact mechanism. What is indisputable is its effectiveness. A reminder is appropriate here that the same puzzle is true of large sectors of Western medicine: many very simple and long-established "cures" have been discovered accidentally, passed down from generation to generation, and elude discovery about exactly why they work.

Tobacco is one of the most powerful stimulants known. Its active ingredient, nicotine, is a deadly toxic chemical. Long before medical science acknowledged that tobacco is habit-forming, smokers knew how hopelessly hooked they were. In some ways, tobacco is even more addictive than "hard" drugs such as heroin. Because it takes only a few seconds for the stimulant to reach brain cells, a regular smoker can indulge in "hits" three or more times an hour, all day long. Small wonder that breaking the habit is so difficult.

Helping people quit smoking has become big business. Television ads tout machines and patent medications that promise to help. Smoking cessation programs run by private clinics number in the hundreds. These programs are generally expensive but have low success rates. And even when they work, it is at the expense of prolonged periods of anxiety and discomfort to the smoker. Acupuncture, on the other hand, offers a safe, relatively inexpensive, and effective route to detoxification.

Approximately 80 percent of those treated with needles give up cigarettes after two to five short sessions. For all addictions, the usual treatment consists of placing fine needles in each external ear. Because there is so little cushiony material in this area, the patient does feel a small pinch at insertion, but always less pain than from a hypodermic needle used for injection or blood removal. There is no pain once the needles are in place, nor is there pain upon removal. A low-level electrical stimulation may be added to enhance the effect. The current is provided by a 9-volt battery system, similar to the charge of a common flashlight. Needles are left in place for fifteen to thirty minutes. Some acupuncturists also needle body points at the same time. Former smokers I have treated offer their evaluations:

"I am mystified by what happened and cannot explain it. I walked out of the office completely cured. I have no desire to smoke, and I loved smoking. It was so much a part of my life that I am amazed to be free of it!"

"It was like a revelation how many of my smoking-related health symptoms disappeared when I stopped."

"I couldn't stand the taste of cigarettes after a couple of treatments. Acupuncture gave me the energy and the mental power to stay stopped."

Alcoholics admit burning themselves out using conventional means to cope with withdrawal. Drugs to combat convulsions, hallucinations, and extreme anxiety can help, but they too can be addictive. Alcohol withdrawal is dangerous and can sometimes cause stroke, heart attack, or other permanent damage. But in clinics where acupuncture has been used to ease detoxification, success has been remarkable.

Two such detox clinics are operating in New York City, one in Brooklyn under Dr. Bernard Bihari, and the other in the Bronx, directed since 1973 by Dr. Michael Smith. The Brooklyn center treats only alcoholics who have been in other detox programs and so provides a way to compare acupuncture to other treatments.

The Bronx clinic offers acupuncture therapy and herbal remedies along with counseling to walk-ins and stayovers in its detox center. It reports a 90 percent success rate in relieving acute withdrawal symptoms and persuading alcoholics to continue treatment. It estimates that 60 percent of those who receive the recommended series of treatments over a two-week program remain alcohol-free for at least several months. The Bronx clinic receives about a 110 new patients a day.

Another model program has been established on the Crow and Sioux American Indian reservations. In the summer of 1987, the National Acupuncture Detoxification Association sponsored training in these communities for Native American staff workers in alcoholism programs. More than 150 acupuncture treatments were conducted at several sites. Tribal leaders observed the process and were convinced by the results. Acupuncture was an answer to urgent health needs on the reservations.

Some of the Indian staff members learned ear acupuncture well enough to provide regular treatment. Needling was so successful that the need for accompanying detox drugs was decreased. When people experience victories in an early stage of withdrawal, they are encouraged to continue. The results were so promising that the U.S. Indian Health Service in Aberdeen, South Dakota, is considering a similar program for the Mohawk reservation, as well as an acupuncture treatment center to serve the entire region.

One of the country's first alcohol detox studies was done in Hennepin County Detox Center, in Minneapolis. A group of fifty-four hardcore alcoholic recidivists were chosen to determine if sobriety could be achieved and episodes of drinking or admissions to detox could be decreased by acupuncture. Acupuncture treatments were given to twenty-seven patients and the other twenty-five made up the control group. The mean number of years of alcohol abuse was around twenty.

Significant differences were noted between treatment and control patients. The completion rate was significantly higher for treatment group patients than control group patient. The control group expressed a significantly stronger need for alcohol than did those in the treatment group. As the study progressed, the frequency of drinking episodes and detox admissions was clearly apparent and significantly higher in the control group. Treatment patients stated that acupuncture therapy had decreased their desire to drink.[6]

The Bronx center also treats drug addicts with acupuncture and without methadone. In 1979 Dr. Smith found methadone withdrawal to be even harsher than heroin detoxification. In addition, methadone has been linked to bone deterioration, liver damage, insomnia, and anxiety. Methadone works by suppressing normal physical feelings and sensations, not just the drug withdrawal symptoms alone. It produces a kind of "maintenance high," which is itself addictive. Many practitioners in conventional drug abuse programs come to see themselves as custodial suppliers of drugs that ease withdrawal. It is as if they have themselves become drug-pushers. And when patients complain of continuing problems with anxiety and depression, they are told, "You just have to be strong and endure it." The immediate effects of giving up a drug—even with the help of the limited support provided by a program—are often so overwhelming that addicts find it preferable to give up the program rather than the drug. These programs are expensive to operate, and long waiting lists discourage addicts from signing up.

Acupuncture therapy programs treat withdrawal separately from the addiction. Patients are initially needled daily for five to nine days, and twice daily if necessary for depression, insomnia, or persistent craving. After this regimen, most are drug-free. Addicts who suffer a relapse can be needled again promptly. These patients go on to counseling and other self-help programs.

Both Drs. Smith and Bihari have found acupuncture helpful in treating crack addicts. In a clinical survey of one thousand five hundred patients treated with acupuncture and psychological and social intervention, clients find it easier to become and remain drug-free.[7]

"The technique," say Drs. Smith and Bihari, "though not a panacea for addiction, is the most helpful thing I've seen yet." Detoxing with acupuncture is safe, inexpensive, and simple. Because it can be accomplished in any setting, an addict need not remain on a long waiting list to enter expensive facilities. Moreover, acupuncture can deal with more than one addiction at a time, what is sometimes called "cross-addiction." Persons who are dependent on alcohol plus valium or even "hard" drugs can have their dual addictions treated simultaneously. Similarly, patients who have unwittingly become dependent on one of the drugs commonly used by psychiatrists (librium or valium, for example) can break their addiction through needling. New Mexico has become the first state to adopt acupuncture in its detoxification programs. Clinics have been opened in five cities to provide acupuncture to nearly half of the state's six hundred registered drug abusers. The cost is estimated to be one-tenth that of conventional methadone programs.

Anyone who has even tried to lose weight knows how stressful it is. There are swings from guilt to anger to anxiety. Discouragement, self-hatred, and a general feeling of low self-worth are the experiences of millions of Americans who try one kind of diet after another. If there is some small weight loss, the weight is usually regained at a later date, only to start the cycle anew. Acupuncture helps to make weight loss less stressful and more permanent by curbing the appetite. It is simple: you eat less because you are not constantly hungry. Patients lose weight slowly, steadily, and healthfully—without starvation that shocks the system. The body's metabolism readjusts to improved eating habits. The patient eats normal fare, just less of it, without being deprived of occasional treats, and so the food craving goes away.

Treatment begins with a look at the patient's body and eating habits. Problems with constipation, indigestion, and gas and fluid retention receive attention. Restoring these imbalances helps weight loss to occur. Patients report that their food cravings for fats, sweets, and carbohydrates are curbed; they simply eat less without having to think about it. Obsessions with food are lifted.

Needling takes place at body or ear points; the exact locations are determined by the needs of each person. I personally like to place a small magnet-type earring in the external ear for the patient to wear between sessions. This device constantly stimulates the appetite center of the brain, reminding it to "take it easy" while the subject goes about his daily routine. Most patients begin to lose about two pounds per week as treatment continues.

Addictions are poorly understood. For years researchers have been searching for some evidence of genetic predispositions to alcoholism and other substance abuse patterns. Whatever the underlying reasons why one person becomes an addict and another doesn't, the effects are the same. The addicted person becomes dependent on a substance, and the body requires it in regular doses. These substances are usually toxic and can do great damage. But addicts must have the substance or else they will go into physical withdrawal. In the case of alcoholics, the central nervous system receives such a shock when alcohol is abruptly denied that delirium tremens (DTs) may result, characterized by visual and/or auditory hallucinations, epileptic-like convulsions, profuse sweating, nausea, and insomnia. This is why users administer themselves "maintenance doses" rather than face withdrawal. Addicts to heroin and other drugs say that they must have their daily minimum fix just to stay "normal"; they have long ceased to experience the pleasurable high the drugs once produced. Acupuncture can eliminate withdrawal symptoms. The body and nervous system do not go into shock when the drink, nicotine, or drug is removed. Once withdrawal is completed, the patient can start on the road to living substance-free.

Many former addicts choose some form of counseling or twelve-step program to help them adjust to the new lifestyle made possible by being "clean and dry." They have regained body harmony and need to relearn how to live without dependence. Acupuncture makes it all possible. As one of my patients put it, "I don't know how or why acupuncture works, but it absolutely, positively works!"

NOTES

1. Gu Yueshan, et al. "Observation on 473 Cases of Weight Reduction Treated by Implanting Seeds at Ear Points." *Chinese Acupuncture and Moxibustion.* 8 (1): 15-16, 1988.
2. V. N. Zalesskiy. "Laser Acupuncture Reduces Cigarette Smoking: A Preliminary Report." *Acupuncture and Electrotherapy Research.* 8: 297-302, 1983.
3. J. A. Newmeyer, G. Johnson, S. Klot. Acupuncture as a Detoxification Modality." *Journal of Psychoactive Drugs.* 16 (3): 241-261, 1984.
4. Ralph Allen Dale. "Addictions and Acupuncture: The Treatment Methods, Formulae, Effectiveness and Limitations." *American Journal of Acupuncture.* 21 (3): 247-263, 1993.
5. R. J. Kroening, T. D. Oleson. "Rapid Narcotic Detoxification in Chronic Pain Patients Treated with Auricular Electroacupuncture and Naloxone." *International Journal of Addictions.* 20 (9): 1347-1360, 1985.
6. Milton L. Bullock, Andrew J. Umen, Patricia D. Culliton, Robert T. Olander. "Acupuncture Treatment of Alcohol Recidivism: A Pilot Study." *American Journal of Acupuncture.* 15 (4): 313-320, 1987.
7. Michael O. Smith. "Acupuncture Treatment for Crack: Clinical Survey of 1,500 Patients Treated." *American Journal of Acupuncture.* 16 (3): 241-247, 1988.

REFERENCES

Historical and clinical information on drug addictions can be found in many issues of *The American Journal of Acupuncture*. Several informative ones are M. O. Smith, et al., "Acupuncture Treatment of Drug Addiction and Alcohol Abuse" (vol. 10, No. 2, 1982), M. O. Smith, et al., "Detoxification in a Drug and Alcohol Abuse Treatment Setting" (vol. 12, no. 3, 1984), and M. L. Bullock, et al., "Acupuncture Treatment of Alcohol Recidivism: A Pilot Study" (vol. 15, no. 4, 1985).

Chapter 16

ACUPUNCTURE AND MENTAL HEALTH

The psychiatrist Dr. Leon Hammer reflects that "acupuncture fit well into the framework of a humanistic psychotherapeutic tradition, and many patients, especially those coming only for physical problems, frequently opened up to their deepest, unexpressed and even unknown feelings and thoughts."[1]

Acupuncture can ready patients for achieving the goal of therapy: change. Depressed persons can begin to accept responsibility for their negativity and embrace joy once again. Obsessive persons become less rigid and start to experience freedom from obsessive acts. Schizoid persons learn to recognize their detachment as an obstacle to wellness. Schizophrenic persons begin to reassemble the fragmented parts of their selves. And paranoid persons are able to look within themselves to find the causes of their unhappiness.

Again and again we see patients discover themselves through acupuncture. They become aware of their bodies and confront the tensions, rigidities, pains, and physical discomforts caused by their own thoughts and actions. Above all, acupuncture helps people develop an awareness of their psyches—the emotions, memories, dreams, and ideas they have lived with all their lives. And acupuncture patients experience a newfound feeling of well-being and self-healing. They began to feel truly alive.

When patients first experience release from depression, pain, and stress, they also start to realize that further relief is possible. It is the beginning of hope. As their health gradually improves, they realize that they don't have to accept the accustomed misery of life. It is inspiring and enlightening to listen to patients talk about these changes; they speak of awareness, balance, a feeling of self-worth. Their newfound energy has given them strength and unsuspected resources to cope. Patients recovering from depression describe a rejuvenated capacity to communicate and relate to others, heightened satisfaction with life, and a growing spirituality.

Acupuncture profoundly affects psychophysiological afflictions. Two years ago, I took on the case of a formerly homeless woman. She had lived on the streets for more than a decade with mental illness and an alcohol problem. Before I met her, she had voluntarily entered a rehabilitation facility. When she came to me, she was part of an outpatient daily rehab program that provided counseling and occupational therapy. She had physical problems, including colitis, migraine headaches, back and leg pain, and peripheral neuropathy (diminished circulation in her legs). She also had what we practitioners call "disturbed spirit" problems: anxiety, fear, low self-esteem, insomnia, palpitations, and dizziness. It was inspiring to observe the changes that took place with needling sessions. Her physical problems disappeared, leaving her the strength to set goals, such as returning to school and finding a job. She felt mentally more in control as she began to talk about and act on long-range plans for her life. At our final meeting, she thanked me for all that the acupuncture had done for her. "I have come out of a very black room," she said, "and I see myself standing on the threshold of a new life. It's scary, but it's also wonderful."

Early Traditional Chinese Medicine practitioners concentrated on the processes of disease. They gathered subtle signals and symptoms indicating early signs of breakdown in health, and they catalogued and codified their observations. They viewed disease as a process that begins with vague and sometimes unclear messages from the body. Of course, these early practitioners recognized and were acquainted with gross pathologies and the wide range of visible, acute disease. But it was the subtle and less objective and concrete aspects of disease that often intrigued them. We practitioners must deal with the observable features of the body and its systems, but we look deeper to discover the underlying, less readily tangible force that animates all of these systems.

When the life force flows smoothly, health flourishes; when the life force is blocked, sickness prevails. A practitioner's job is to return the energy flow to normal and keep it there. The Chinese medical model has the conceptual tools to explain the relationships between the psyche and the body and to correct imbalances between the two. Any active factor, whether human or environmental, that interferes with the life force will push the body and mind to the disease end of the spectrum. I touched on these philosophical/medical views of TCM in Chapter 3, in which I discussed yin/yang, the concept of Chi and so on. The specific factors that cause disease (or health) center around eating, working, sexual functioning, and the emotions. Environmental factors such as weather, climate, exposure to pathogens (disease-causing agents), and pollution also influence health. Using the many diagnostic methods in which we are schooled, we try to ascertain the "what, when, why, and how" of these different factors and the ways they affect the integrity of the person's body and life force.

Acupuncturists are attentive to early signs of disease. Trained to "read" the body, tongue, eyes, and pulse, we can recognize when the body is in the early stages of disruption. Let me give an example. A concert singer came to me after her career stopped abruptly because of her health. Her chief physical complaints were menstrual irregularity, PMS, and severe fear and confusion about her career and future. In her distress, she had sought out conventional physicians who prescribed medications, and she underwent psychotherapy. Months passed with no change, no sign of improvement.

She turned to acupuncture out of mounting fear and frustration. Now, things began to happen. During the needling treatments, she gained insights into her marriage and her career. The sadness and weeping she so often exhibited in early sessions were replaced in later sessions by more positive energy release. She began to speak about reaching into herself and drawing on her inner resources rather than reaching out into the world. Her prolonged depressive episode and sense of defeat resolved. She began to incorporate teaching with performing. She said to me, "I have come to recognize that I have achieved much. It is time to recognize, accept and value my achievement, and to go on to help those coming up. If I can help others do their best, I will have produced much of lasting value."

Negativity, agitation, irritability, withdrawal, and guilt are characteristic symptoms of the disruption of particular channel energies. This spectrum of emotions can inhibit the physical body. Hal, a patient in his 40s, told me, "I used to fidget with my legs, constantly moving them. It didn't matter where I was, or what I was feeling or doing. I was always restless. I have a long history of depression. I'm divorced and have three children. I can't say that I'm particularly tender toward my kids. I guess I can't express love. I'm so frustrated; I see myself holding back all my emotions, good and bad."

When Hal talked about his health, the picture was not much brighter. "I have been on medication and even had shock therapy. I constantly suffer with my stomach; it churns all day long. It feels like I have a big knot in there, and I am nauseous all day long. I really don't feel well. There's a lot of tension in my neck and back too."

Hal described feelings of unhappiness, emotions that rested on feelings of worthlessness and self-deprecation. There was an accompanying physical side to his enduring discomfort—complaints of chronic ill-health. Having won no lasting relief from conventional treatment that included antidepressant drugs, Hal finally consulted me. He recalls the first session vividly: "After the needles were in, I felt the strangest sensations in my stomach. I can't describe it as pain, just a new and very strong feeling." From the first treatment he reported all of the old stomach complaints had ended.

With a few more weekly treatments, the muscle tension in his neck and back went away. Hal reported that he was beginning to visit with his sons more often and that he spent time thinking of what they would enjoy doing. He spoke of them less and less as a source of pressure and aggravation. He began to appear less hurried, less like a man wanting impatiently to get on with something—anything.

Karl, a patient in his mid-30s, had suffered from cyclic depression for years. He said, "For three or four days every month, I could not move. I was irritable, unable to focus on my work or stay alert. For days, I sat in my chair at home, neither happy nor bored nor angry. I was just nothing. Needless to say, I could also be argumentative with everybody and nasty to my wife." Karl was fearful of closeness of any kind. He said that his memories of months at a time were just "missing," and he concluded that he was having a mental breakdown.

Karl detected changes after five acupuncture sessions. "The first month I got through with fewer symptoms," he said. "In the second month

I really noticed changes. I had only one bad day and a couple of blah ones."
As we continued therapy, he was calm enough to, as he said, "begin to take
stock of myself." His renewed energy and interest in life stimulated him
to search for and find a good job. He stated, "I found that I could work with
people much more easily than I had ever remembered. I was definitely less
argumentative, less ready to find fault with everybody, including my wife.
Speaking of her, she is thrilled about the changes. She says I am much
easier to live with now." Karl reported that his general level of well-being
had vastly improved. "On a day-to-day basis, I am positive, do not sleep
so much, have more energy, and am enjoying my life." He now returns for
an occasional treatment, especially when he feels that he is "slipping" into
old patterns.

In a schizophrenic patient I treated, I found a young man unnurtured
by his family and bonded to no one. Jack was a healthy-looking 22-year-
old. Our first interview lasted over two hours because he was unable to
relate information or answer questions easily. He hallucinated about
voices he heard. He did relate that his father had been diagnosed as manic-
depressive, his mother as a schizoid personality, and his brother was
severely depressed. He had a sister on whom he depended for emotional
support. The family had continual bad times, which Jack attributed to his
mother. He would report events such as: "This week my mother broke
three VCRs, one after the other. She just won't learn how to use them right
and gets mad and breaks them." The family's eating habits were erratic.
Asked what they'd had for dinner the previous night, he told me, "my
father came home with three cakes for supper."

Jack had begun engineering school but was forced to drop his
studies because of his "voices." Although he was medicated with some of
the most powerful drugs known, he heard the voices all the time. When he
tried to exercise at the local "Y," if there was a woman in the body-building
area, the voices invariably grew louder and louder, forcing him to leave.
He hoped the acupuncture would still the voices that belittled him and
accused him of having evil thoughts. Ultimately, he hoped to keep his
mental illness in check so that he would not have to be hospitalized.

I gave him his first acupuncture treatment and laid out a program of
herbal medicines and further weekly visits. When he came the next time,
he reported that the voices had gone down 50 percent in volume. Jack had
many more acupuncture sessions, with additional help from nutritional
supplements and herbal medicines. The disabling voices finally disappeared. Jack's thought processes began to be more orderly, and he

prepared to reenter college. He was no longer the acutely fragmented and disorganized young man I'd first encountered.

In China a concerted attempt has been made to integrate traditional treatment with modern psychiatric care. An effort has begun to train health care workers to recognize early stress symptoms, which can then be treated before the patient's condition deteriorates into full-blown disease. Outpatient clinics screen, test, and diagnose patients using both Western and traditional medical methods. Early treatment is done on an outpatient basis primarily through needling and herbal medicines. Because of early intervention, most patients do not require hospital admission.

When a patient does require hospitalization, he enters a highly structured program that integrates therapies. Exercise, occupational work-study activities, acupuncture, herbs, and Western drugs are combined. Herbal medicines and acupuncture treatment enhance the action of medication. Because doctors can prescribe a much lower dosage of drugs than would otherwise be required, the possibility of addiction or long-term adverse effects is lessened. Needling treats both physical and mental symptoms simultaneously. Patients who are in a manic state or who are greatly agitated can be calmed to the point where they can participate in rehabilitation routines. Conversely, depressed and lethargic patients are stimulated and are thereby more receptive to other treatment.

In Chinese hospitals, acupuncture treatments are given twice a day over a three- to four-week period. Sessions last five to twenty minutes. Herbal medicines are administered three or four times a day. The average hospital stay is several months; very few patients require hospitalization for longer periods. There is close followup on the outpatient level after discharge.

China is investing huge sums of money and medical personnel in its effort to cure mental illness. Schizophrenia accounts for 30 to 40 percent of all cases treated. One-third of these cases are acute. When such a case presents itself at the outpatient level, immediate combined therapy is begun. The results are impressive: 55 percent of those ill for six months or less recover in only a few weeks. Western drugs are administered for a short time, while herbal therapy and needling are provided in a long-term program.[2]

Modern scientific studies have tried to explain why acupuncture works so well. Russian researchers on neurosis and depressive disorders found biochemical differences in the blood and urine samples of patients before and after needling.[3] Acupuncture raises specific neurotransmitter and hormone levels, substances that are responsible for subjective feelings of well-being.

Australian researchers studied the efficacy of acupuncture treatment on anxiety and stress-related illnesses and have concluded that acupuncture provides an extremely cost-effective, side effect-free method of dealing with anxiety.[4] Another Australian study concludes that ear acupuncture lowers tension, produces calmness and creates euphoria in treated alcoholics. Eighty-seven percent of patients said their lifestyle, drinking patterns and physical, mental, and social health had changed for the better, and they became more motivated to improve themselves.[5]

In Japan, research has been done on individuals in high-stress occupations, such as taxi-driving. Drivers who showed symptoms of agitation and strain found relief after several weeks of acupuncture sessions.[6] Some clues to this success can be found in the muscular system, the body's first indicator of imbalance. When stress is experienced for a long period of time, tenderness develops at various locations in the body. Some neurologists call these locations "trigger points." Many of these trigger points, in turn, correspond to acupuncture points known for many hundreds of years. Needling them reduces the built-up tension.

Western therapies emphasize the direct, intrusive attack by cutting into the body or introducing powerful chemicals; the assumption is that healing will follow. In contrast, the practitioner of acupuncture believes that the body heals itself, given appropriate outside influence. TCM provides deep, nourishing healing that permits the patient the luxury of feeling progressively stronger and more balanced without dependence on artificial agents. Acupuncture stirs and cultivates the feelings of wellness and lets us feel alive on all levels.

NOTES

1. Leon Hammer, *Dragon Rises—Red Bird Flies: Psychology and Chinese Medicine.* Tarrytown, New York: Station Hill Press, 1990, 18.
2. Shi Zhengxiu. "Treatment of 500 Cases of Schizophrenia by Acupuncture." *Chinese Acupuncture and Moxibustion.* 5 (4): 2-4, 1985.
3. S. E. Poyakov. "Acupuncture in the Treatment of Patients with Endogenic Depression." *Zh. Nevropatol. Psikh.* 87 (4): 604-608, 1987.
4. S. Strauss. "Anxiety and Acupuncture." Second Australian Interna-

tional Congress of Contemporary Acupuncture, Melbourne, October 25-26, 1982. Meeting Paper.
5.   Charles Gall. "Auricular Psychotherapy for Alcohol Addicts." Second Australian International Congress of Contemporary Acupuncture, Melbourne, October 25-29, 1982. Meeting Paper.
6.   M. Ogiwara. "The Effects of Acupuncture on the Health of Taxi Drivers." *Journal of the Japan Society of Acupuncture.* 32 (1): 67-73, 1982.

REFERENCES

A good starting point for reading about mental health in relation to acupuncture is Y. Requera, *Character and Health: The Relationship of Acupuncture and Psychology* (1989). Interesting material on Asian therapies can be found in C. S. Cheung, et al., *Mental Dysfunction as Treated by Traditional Chinese Medicine* (1981), M. Livingston and P. Lowinger, *The Minds of the Chinese People: Mental Health in the New China* (1983), and L. Hammer, *Dragon Rises—Red Bird Flies* (1990).

Part 3

ACUPUNCTURE IN THE UNITED STATES

Chapter 17

THE LEGAL STATUS OF ACUPUNCTURE

There is a "great tradition" in Chinese medicine, and its roots extend back two millennia. This tradition is the cumulation of careful experimentation and has produced a sophisticated body of knowledge about the causes of disease and its diagnosis, treatment, and prevention. As the world shrinks, the American medical model will be forced to recognize Traditional Chinese Medicine.

The American medical establishment has consistently and actively resisted the acceptance of Chinese practices, even though many individual Western doctors have recognized the obvious effectiveness of acupuncture. The claims that Eastern medicine is unsafe, unscientific, and ineffective deny legitimacy to a discipline that has a different theoretical basis and employs different tools and techniques.

Until the 1970s, it was unusual to find acupuncturists in the United States. The term itself was almost unknown. Acupuncture was relegated to the status of a Ripley's "Believe It or Not" novelty in the popular press. Only a small number of Americans who had lived and traveled in the Far

East had any acquaintance with Chinese medicine or had any exposure to it. Most Americans, once they found that it entailed being stuck with needles, probably would have shied away from it.

After World War II, rumors about acupuncture began to cross the English Channel from France, where it had been used for decades (see Chapter 14). When a London women's magazine published an article on the subject, the editors received over ten thousand requests for more information. The public was interested and ready to try it.

Here in the United States we must suspend judgment and disregard those who argue against acupuncture because of its unfamiliar and unorthodox procedures. These holdouts steadfastly ignore the fact that acupuncture is the standard form of medicine for one-third of the world's population. In China, millions of people are needled daily for all kinds of health problems; the overall cure rate is 90 percent.[1] In Japan, Great Britain, and Canada, the success rates are 83 percent, 70 percent and 80 percent, respectively.[2, 3, 4]

There are obvious fallacies and inconsistencies in the position that acupuncture is ineffective and unsafe and lacks scientific foundation. Over the last thirty years we have come to know more about the mechanics and workings of acupuncture than we know about the mechanics of many well-accepted western practices. For example, Western medical thinking ignores the fact that the majority of "trigger points" accepted and used by Western physicians and physiotherapists correlate with acupuncture points.

The criticism that acupuncture is ineffective ignores extensive evidence of its clinical success. Moreover, in a typical clinical situation, the acupuncturist receives the conventional physician's failures. People who have had no results from accepted conventional practice seek out alternatives in desperation.

The status and practice of acupuncture in this country are vague, contradictory, and ill defined. Some Western doctors have begun to accept it piecemeal: they are willing to acknowledge that needling helps with pain or addictions, but they will not accept the practice in general. In the face of such intolerance, it is unrealistic to think that acupuncture will be fully accepted in the near future. The burden of proof that the practice is risky, ineffective, and scientifically unsound, however, rests on the American medical establishment.

In the 1980 landmark case of *Andrews v. Ballard*, the U.S. District Court of the Southern District of Texas held that the right to receive acupuncture is a fundamental personal right. The court concluded that the

Texas Medical Practice Act, which regulates the practice of medicine in that state, had unconstitutionally interfered with the citizen's right to privacy.

The *Andrews* case was a class action suit brought by forty-six persons who either had obtained or wanted to obtain acupuncture treatment. The plaintiffs argued that the right to receive acupuncture treatment is among those personal rights deemed fundamental. Texas statute thus deprived citizens of a constitutional right of privacy founded in the due process clause of the fourteenth amendment, which encompasses the decision to obtain or reject medical treatment because it limited the practice of acupuncture to physicians only. Judgment on the case noted that the decision to receive acupuncture treatment clearly meets the statutory criteria of "important," because good health profoundly affects life, and "personal," because it involved an individual's body.

The determination that the plaintiffs had a right to receive acupuncture treatment is the most important aspect of the case. The *Andrews* case was a balanced scale between the fundamental right of an individual to receive acupuncture treatment and the state's legitimate interest in preserving the health and safety of the public by regulating the practice of medicine. The court found that due to the apparent safety and effectiveness of acupuncture, the "physicians only" requirement was unnecessary. The court further found that in those states that allow nonphysician practice of acupuncture, a potential misdiagnosis or complication could be averted by requiring either a consultation and diagnosis with a physician prior to treatment by acupuncture.

The court rejected argument on the grounds that the Medical Practice Act, in total self-contradiction, prohibited the formally trained acupuncturist from practicing while allowing the admittedly untrained but medically licensed physician to practice acupuncture. Doctors could needle without having to establish that they had learned the skills necessary to do so. Texas medical schools do not teach acupuncture, and licensing examinations do not test for proficiency in acupuncture.

Finally, the court acknowledged that complications during needling are highly unlikely, but it established the requirement that acupuncturists pass a course on emergency medical treatment (EMT) or make arrangements to have EMT available. This requirement would protect the patient without interfering with his constitutional rights. Thus, the court concluded that the "physicians only" restriction had the practical effect of making acupuncture unavailable in the state of Texas, leaving the patient no choice except conventional medicine. It thus violated the patient's fundamental right to choose how best to relieve pain and suffering.

The Texas judgment aside, acupuncture has had a discouraging legal history in the United States. Many states have no rulings at all, and among those states that do, there is a wide range of opinion as to how acupuncture is to be practiced. In some states, acupuncturists are allowed to work only in a medical doctor's office, under direct supervision. This physician may, in turn, supervise only one Traditional Chinese Medicine practitioner. To ensure that the supervising doctor has sufficient understanding of the procedures involved, he must document training in acupuncture. In any given state, only a few physicians will have received basic instruction in needling, and even those few will lack the qualifications of a well-trained acupuncturist. This places great restrictions on the general availability of acupuncture therapy. Not many medical doctors are willing to spend the requisite time learning a technique about which they are skeptical in the first place.

A small number of states require prospective patients to obtain a referral from a licensed physician before they can receive acupuncture treatment. Many patients are unable to obtain referrals because they must seek out one of the few doctors willing to comply; much inconvenience and expense may therefore be involved. Referral requirements interfere with the patient's right to decide on appropriate medical treatment and may, in fact, be unconstitutional. The matter has not yet been decided in the courts.

Inconsistencies in the requirements to practice acupuncture abound. In some states, a physician with six months' training is considered to be an acupuncturist. Yet the same policy considers the nonphysician with three years' formal and rigorous schooling to be no more than an "acupuncture assistant" similar to a paramedical assistant. And some states allow only an M.D. to practice acupuncture. This is like allowing a dentist to practice as a heart surgeon simply because he has a medical degree.

Discrimination and outright harassment plague the nonphysician practitioner. In 1981 the American Medical Association declared that acupuncture is eminently respectable as long as it is performed by a physician. This implies that the extensive and time-honored training of TCM practitioners is inferior to the untrained skills of an establishment member. Of course, the refusal to protect the public by allowing untrained physicians to perform acupuncture derives from the arrogant assumption that Western medical training is adequate preparation for acupuncture practice. State regulations limiting acupuncture practice to physicians favor Western medicine and deny that acupuncture is a complete medical modality. There are no grounds, scientific or otherwise, for excluding qualified people from practicing Chinese medicine simply because they do not also qualify to practice Western medicine.

One frequent justification for curtailing acupuncture in this country is the need to protect the public from certain perceived risks such as breaking needles or fainting patients. Insofar as these are possibilities, albeit remote ones, the risk would be best eliminated by requiring acupuncturists to undergo EMT training. If acupuncturists are EMT qualified, a medical degree is superfluous for any minor mishap.

Another reason given for requiring medical supervision is that it may prevent patients from receiving acupuncture for conditions whose underlying cause requires Western medical treatment—a case of cardiac arrest or acute appendicitis, for instance. This rationale is also unwarranted. There is no evidence of inappropriate treatment replacing conventional care in states where unsupervised practice is permitted. The opposite is true. The great majority of acupuncture patients seek needling therapy as a last resort, after having received innumerable and often contradictory Western diagnoses and after having undergone expensive, prolonged, and ineffective Western medical treatment.

At the federal level, little attention is given to the availability and regulation of acupuncture. FDA guidelines were adopted in 1972 on the basis of consensus reached at a one-day invitational conference that year and have never been updated. This meeting was attended largely by members of the medical profession whose experience with acupuncture was nonexistent. The conference did not investigate the merits of acupuncture. It merely issued a position paper on the labeling of devices like acupuncture needles and electro-acupuncture machines. No effort was made to evaluate the safety and effectiveness of the acupuncture therapy itself.

At present, policies regarding acupuncture are blatantly exclusionary to nonphysician practitioners, and patients' testimony on behalf of acupuncture is persistently belittled by the medical community. The United States needs one good model to emulate. Perhaps the licensing laws in Nevada come the closest to informed, rational regulation. In 1973 the state passed a comprehensive acupuncture law following vigorous lobbying by patients and a month-long series of demonstrations of acupuncture, during which Dr. Yee-Rung Lok needled hundreds of people, including several Nevada state legislators.

Nevada state law regards Eastern medicine as separate and distinct from its Western counterpart and sets up special administrative machinery to govern its practice. Doctors, along with chiropractors and physical therapists, are not automatically qualified to practice acupuncture in Nevada. Any M.D. wishing to become an acupuncture specialist must obtain licensing from the State Board of Oriental Medicine. A five-member board administers the law, examines applicants, and grants licenses. To obtain a license, one must have studied at an accredited institution for four years, have interned for six years, and have passed a state-approved examination. Such an environment sanctions practitioners with valued skills and notifies the patient-consumer that he is in safe hands.

NOTES

1.   *Chinese Medical Journal*, September 1981.
2.   Yoshio Oshima. "A View of the Past and Present of Acupuncture Medicine and Future Prospects." *Journal of the Japan Society of Acupuncture*. 36 (3): 143-151, 1986.
3.   G. T. Lewith, D. Machin. "On the Evaluation of the Clinical Effects of Acupuncture." *Pain*. 16 (2): 111-127, 1983.
4.   L. M. Rapson. "Acupuncture: A Useful Treatment Modality." *Canadian Family Physician*. 30 (1): 109-115, 1984.

REFERENCES

For a thorough review of the legal status of acupuncture, see the article by Ginger McRae, "A Critical Review of U. S. Acupuncture Regulation" in *American Journal of Acupuncture* (vol. 10, no. 4, 1982), or Paul A. Drummond's "The Decision for Acupuncture Treatment: An Expansion of the Right of Privacy" in *American Journal of Acupuncture* (vol. 10, no. 3, 1982).

Chapter 18

THE FUTURE OF ACUPUNCTURE

Most Americans mistakenly believe that conventional medicine is the only sound and legitimate choice. In this country, doctors and hospitals enjoy a monopoly on the kinds of medicine that are practiced. Newspapers, magazines, books, and television announce the latest medical breakthroughs, but only in the area of conventional drugs or surgery. Little mainstream reporting is done on alternative medicine. But there are other medical options, equally respectable, equally well founded, and scientifically and clinically proven. There is growing and indisputable evidence that alternative treatment based on Traditional Chinese Medicine works. And it is less intrusive, safer, and much cheaper.

The nation's annual health bill comes to many billions of dollars. Yet Americans do not seem to have purchased better health. In his book, *Male Practice: How Doctors Manipulate Women*, Dr. Robert Mendelsohn observes: "The question that worries me, and should worry you, won't be answered until we discover the long-term effects of the radical pharmaceutical and surgical interventions of recent decades . . ."[1]

In Britain, information on the health of its citizens is routinely included in the government's statistical surveys. Shockingly, over half of all men and nearly three-quarters of all women reported that they suffered from chronic health problems. In round figures, this means that half the population considered themselves chronically ill, and one-quarter of the population was constantly preoccupied with the special care they needed because of poor health.[2]

In Australia, sample surveys found that only eleven percent of those interviewed had no injury, illness, or disability to report.

In the United States, a one-year health care expenditure study reported that over sixty percent of the American population had prescriptions filled. Any examination of the state of sickness and health of the populations in developed countries raises the concern that despite the enormous growth of prescriptions drugs, the benefits are elusive.[3]

When we consider that the average hospital patient in the United States is given eight or more different drugs, the possibilities of adverse reactions and rates of iatrogenesis (doctor-caused disease) are important issues. Monitoring adverse reactions had been an ongoing project of the Boston Collaborative Drug Surveillance Program started by Dr. Herscel Jick. Dr. Jick reported that about one out of three hospitalized patients suffered adverse effects. In eighty percent of these cases, the reactions were rated moderate or severe. The adverse effects were, in the study's estimation, probably or definitely drug related.[4]

The costs involved in prescription drug reactions and disease are staggering. As far back as 1967, the FDA stated that one and a half million hospitalizations annually were attributed to adverse reactions to drugs. Drug-induced deaths are difficult to determine, but it has been estimated that more people are killed each year by prescribed drugs than by highway accidents.[5] Sociologist David Makofsky comments that "Thirty thousand Americans die yearly from faulty prescriptions, and ten times that number suffer dangerous side effects." He concludes that "American citizens spend more money on medical care than the people of any nation in the world. But we do not receive the best care."[6]

I am not suggesting that doctors put away their drugs and stop performing surgery. I do question why more experiments and studies have not been done to compare the results obtained from drugs and surgery with alternative procedures. Does coronary bypass surgery prolong life and restore better health than would acupuncture, herbal medicine, stress reduction, dietary changes, and exercise programs? Would not some combination of these approaches be superior? If the medical establishment continues to have its way, we may never know.

We could be at a turning point in our medical care history. Discontent with our health care system is widespread, and national debate about how to reorder our health care priorities has become heated. Perhaps we can help shape the future of medical care in this country by examining how alternative medicine has been integrated into programs adopted abroad.

Many countries seem more open to admitting health care alternatives than ours. The government of the Netherlands, for example, has published an extraordinary report by the Commission of Alternative Systems of Medicine showing that 20 percent of the Dutch population has consulted with a practitioner of alternative medicine. The public is no longer uniformly in support of an entrenched medical establishment that allows only its own members to provide health care. In fact, the Commission found that current laws are being broken a thousand times a day by people exercising the freedom to choose their own treatments. When conventional medicine has failed, patients have been finding relief in practices such as acupuncture, especially for the treatment of chronic disease.

The Commission recommends government support of public education about alternative medicine. It also advises financial support to schools that teach alternative medicine, and it proposes establishing a Health Insurance Funds Council for administering insurance reimbursement for alternative medical care. Finally, the Commission acknowledges that most physicians are still antagonistic to competing alternative practices, but concludes that this antagonism is based more on sociopolitical reasons—loss of income, status, and power—than on scientific reasons. It calls for an end to this shortsightedness and encourages greater research, cross-referral, and other kinds of cooperation.

In England doctors themselves are beginning to see medicine differently. A recent survey of British medical students training to become general practitioners found that 81 percent of them wished to receive training in alternative medicine, including hypnosis, acupuncture, and homeopathy. Of practicing British doctors, 21 percent reported that they regularly used at least one alternative procedure. More than one-third of the doctors had referred patients to acupuncture practitioners. The report concluded that, in general, present undergraduate and graduate training does not meet the interests and needs of many physicians.[7]

Since 1972 the Ludwig Boltzman Institute in Vienna, Austria, has served as a training school for physicians, a research laboratory, and a patient care provider in the field of acupuncture. In the first ten years of its existence, one hundred thousand patients were treated. Depending on the illness involved, 66 to 82 percent of all cases were treated successfully. In the same decade, over fifteen thousand physicians and veterinarians from more than a hundred nations received instruction at the Institute.

Research at the Institute establishes acupuncture as an alternative treatment for problems and diseases of the neurological, endocrine, circulatory and muscular systems. Because of the Institute's scientific and clinical work, acupuncture has become integrated into the nation's medical system. Under the socialized medicine of Austria, patients are treated free of charge. Acupuncturists in the city-run hospital clinics treat about sixty-five patients every morning and are always booked many months in advance.

Finland is also integrating acupuncture into its medical curriculum. The goal is to give every medical student a basic knowledge of acupuncture and to supplement Western medical treatment with acupuncture therapy. In a position paper, the government concludes that

> After these eight years of teaching acupuncture in the medical schools of Finland, it is clear that we need alternative medicine for many reasons. Some of the first priorities are: to reduce drug consumption; to lessen the ever increasing costs of modern technical and, in some ways, inhumane medicine; to make available a holistic approach to in-patient care. Finnish experience supports the World Health Organization's view on acupuncture: acupuncture should be integrated with Western Medicine.

Finally, we could learn much from the world's largest medical establishment. In China seven hundred million people use acupuncture as a major component of their health maintenance. One traditional medicine hospital in Beijing, for instance, treats about 2 million outpatients in a single year. A successful joining of Western and Eastern practices results in benefits to all patients.

One example of this cooperation between Eastern and Western medicines can be seen in the treatment of bone fractures. After an initial examination, the limb is set in willow twig splints instead of a plaster cast. The flexible splint allows access for acupuncture and the application of herbal salves and for passive movement. The nature of the break is established through modern X-rays, and an adaptation of the traditional bone-setting technique is used. Needling keeps the avenues of energy and blood flow open above and below the break. Blood circulation is improved, excess interstitial fluid is absorbed, and dead tissue is cleansed away. Herbal plasters applied externally and herbs taken internally speed the healing of the break. Pioneer work in this radical approach toward bone mending was monitored by Tientsin Hospital in over seven hundred cases, all of which healed better and recovered up to 50 percent faster than with the use of cast techniques. This approach eliminates the need for physical therapy and requires minimal to no-drug therapy. The coordinated Western-Eastern method has now become a standard model of treatment in Chinese orthopedic clinics.

Here in the United States, few doctors have given acupuncture its due. But those who work extensively with the therapy accord it high praise. One such physician is Dr. Primitivo Cruz, who treated 573 chronic pain patients over a four-year period at Chenango Memorial Hospital in Norwich, New York. His cases included a wide variety of pain locations, with many underlying causes. In his experience, 60 percent of cases showed 75 to 100 percent improvement. Another 16 percent of cases showed good recovery of 50 percent or more.

Dr. Cruz states: "It is lamentable that up to this time the American Medical Association still considers acupuncture an experimental procedure. It is also most unfair that various hospitals and pain clinics in the country are using transcutaneous neurostimulators in the relief of pain and call the practice 'electric medicine' while this type of procedure is nothing but a variation of electric acupuncture using local points rather than meridian points."[8] One of the more celebrated instances of using what is essentially acupuncture—but calling it something else—was the treatment of President John F. Kennedy's back pain by Dr. Janet Travell. She used "trigger point analgesia," injecting anesthetic by needle at appropriate points, and wrote that the technique worked even when there was no drug in the needle.

Alternative medicines are not routinely available in the United States. I have described some programs that are being adopted in other countries and that may be eventually implemented in this country. In the meantime, what can you do if you become ill? If you are sick and the problem seems to require more than the usual bedrest and chicken soup, of course, you must seek help.

The key is to become informed and stay informed. First, you must know the exact nature of your illness. Western-trained medical professionals have sophisticated equipment and testing procedures to make a tentative diagnosis. Once a diagnosis has been carefully explained to you, the next step is to have all of the treatment options presented in detail. What is proposed: drugs, surgery, physical therapy? Some combination of these, perhaps including dietary change? You must ask in detail what the drawbacks of each plan of action are: what are the possible side effects, both mild and serious? What are the long-term benefits and liabilities? What is the success rate of the various treatments proposed? Above all, what will your quality of life be after conventional treatment?

Next, you should investigate alternative methods of treating your condition before making a choice. Aside from immediately life-threatening crises brought on by sudden disease, accident, or other trauma, there are always alternatives to conventional medicine. You can seek out these alternatives and use them exclusively or in conjunction with conventional treatment. Even if a condition is life-threatening, there are alternatives that can enhance whatever conventional procedures you are undergoing.

At some point in your investigations, you may wish to consult with your doctor about alternative treatments. This is usually disappointing. A majority of physicians in this country know nothing about acupuncture (or any alternative medicine); it will be like talking to a plumber about your electric problems. If your doctor is poorly informed, the response may take one of three forms.

A few physicians will be open-minded and concerned exclusively with your welfare. They will be pleased if you find some method of treatment that benefits you. They will not ridicule or discourage your action and, in rare cases, they may participate in it.

More likely, doctors may become angry or impatient when patients suggest trying an alternative to their own recommendations. Many people realize this in advance, and therefore often do not tell their physician they are exploring alternatives. I have had patients say to me, "Oh, I could never tell my doctor I came here; he would be upset." Other patients say, "Even though you fixed me up, I never told my doctor I went to an acupuncturist, and so he thinks that he cured me!" Or patients who come to me against their doctor's advice, report that "I asked my doctor about acupuncture because nothing seemed to be working for me. Dr. 'Joe' told me that acupuncture was expensive, was just temporary if it worked at all, and if it did work, it was just all in my head."

Doctors may try a kind of sabotage if they learn that you have seen an acupuncturist. Doctors with no knowledge of acupuncture often state categorically that needling will not help your condition. They predict dire results if you are "foolish" enough to try something different. Patients often tell me, "I asked my doctor about trying acupuncture, and he said it would never help. Therefore I must not waste my time on it."

When you tell a doctor you wish to pursue an alternative treatment plan, you are in effect asking him to relinquish some of the power he holds over your personal affairs. It is not uncommon for a doctor to recommend that you see a psychiatrist rather than an acupuncturist, thus giving you the message that your judgment about your health is not to be trusted.

Sometimes doctors make libelous statements about acupuncture practitioners, accusing us of conscious, deliberate fraud. Some doctors have accused us of secretly putting medicines on our needles to achieve results; this is a patent untruth. They also tell patients that needles are unsafe and unsterile and transmit all sorts of disease. These lies are aimed at keeping patients from taking the first step in seeking help outside of the established medical order.

You do have choices. There are a number of possible courses, depending on your problem. First, you can replace conventional treatment entirely with alternatives such as TCM. The management of arthritis is an example. Acupuncture and herbal medicine as a substitute for drugs can manage the pain and inflammation. An exercise program and dietary change can help the body cope with the problem and slow down the rate of degenerative change. With such a strategy you not only would get relief, but also you would not risk long-term organ damage that drugs can cause.

Another possibility arises when you have been ill and have experienced disappointing results from conventional care. A point comes when it is recommended that your treatment be escalated, perhaps with additional drugs or intrusive surgery. This is the time to stop and ask whether acupuncture may work in place of or in conjunction with your present treatment. Osteoarthritis is a case in point. In one study, the pain-reducing effect obtained with acupuncture increased with very session, compared to the therapeutic effects of a new drug (Piroxicam), whose benefits did not increase after two weeks of treatment. In addition to better results, acupuncture was superior to the drug because it had no side effects.[9]

Such a combined therapy approach is now being used successfully in many countries for chronic diseases such as aplastic anemia, hypertension, chronic nephritis, ulcers, diabetes, bronchial asthma, and migraine headache.

People who feel unwell but who have not been able to secure a diagnosis from conventional practitioners can benefit from Traditional Chinese Medicine. A physician who is confronted with contradictory symptoms or ill-defined complaints often finds himself in the dark. He may not be sure which tests to order or how to interpret them. At such times a physician says, "I can't find anything definitely wrong. Let's wait and see how you feel later on." He is telling you that you are not sick enough for him to recognize pathology and that you should come back when things get a lot worse. While this may be a reasonable strategy for treating an automobile, it will not do for a body. You know or sense that something is wrong. This is the time to consult an acupuncturist who is trained in reading and evaluating seemingly unrelated and vague symptoms.

I described our diagnostic procedures earlier: we assemble information in ways that Western physicians cannot in order to piece together a picture of your total body functioning. What may seem to be a minor problem may indeed be the warning of some more serious disease state in the future. As an illustration, a young businessman named Paul came to me because he had not felt well for a long time. His doctor had been no help. Paul complained of intermittent headaches and different kinds of indigestion—from pain to nausea—that seemed unrelated to diet. He wasn't sick enough to be labeled with a known disease, yet he was not well either. In the short span of three treatments, his body underwent a complete change. All of his discomfort was gone, and he felt healthier than he had remembered feeling in a long time.

Finally, TCM can and should be a part of your primary health care even if you are not ill. One of acupuncture's greatest strengths is its preventive effectiveness. We do not hesitate to keep our cars tuned and give them preventive maintenance; we ought to take equally good care of our bodies. Your acupuncturist can provide you with similar insurance.

To be truly preventive, medical intervention has to begin before a disease becomes a pathological reality. Western preventive medicine, with its tests and theories, can tell us that we already have a disease, although it may be in its early states. The term *subclinical* is sometimes used to describe such borderline conditions. But Western doctors admit that, by the time they find these early signs and label them, we are already in a disease state. On the other hand, Traditional Chinese Medicine is capable of distinguishing and identifying even slight deviations from a standard of health. We are alert to the process of deviation before it manifests itself as pathology. We can relate early signs and symptoms to their causes and act to prevent more serious developments.

Two studies in the areas of cardiovascular disease, hyperlipidemia (excessive quantities of fat in the blood) and obesity, support a claim of prevention. The authors of one study applied acupuncture treatment to subjects who had cardiovascular disease complicated with hyperlipidemia. After a total of thirty-six treatments the hemolipoid level decreased dramatically. The results of the other study showed a good therapeutic effect on obesity along with a benign regulatory effect on lipid metabolism and high-density lipoprotein (HDL) cholesterol.[10,11]

Aging and the prevention of senility is an area of current research in TCM. One experiment treating senile dementia with acupuncture and acu-point injection showed a success rate of 42.85 percent and an improvement rate of 42.86 percent. The ratings were based on the results of administered tests (the revised Hasegawa Dementia Scale and the Functional Activity Questionnaire).[12] A second experiment with aging rats reversed movement disorders, as shown in swimming tests, and restored irregular estrus cycles.[13]

Of course, evidence of cancer prevention is widely sought in many research projects. Japanese researchers working with animal studies have shown that acupuncture does have an effect on sarcomas (cancerous tumors). In two studies, the growth of the tumor was significantly inhibited by acupuncture. The possible mechanism being considered is an increase in beta-endorphin and its stimulation of T helper cells or other immune-system cells. In these experiments, the weight of the animals' thymus glands increased. The thymus is essential in the production and maturation of T cells. The researchers also observed an increase in natural antibody values and a prolonged period of increased antibody activity in the body. The researchers believe that immune responses played a large part in the inhibition of cancer cells.[14, 15]

These and other suggestive studies put acupuncture in the forefront of preventive medical alternatives. The best course you can take to safeguard your health is to establish a long-term, familiar relationship with a practitioner of TCM who knows your unique body balances well and can quickly tell when things are not as they should be. Seeing an acupuncturist regularly to talk over your health concerns, having a TCM exam, having a reading of your pulses, and discussing preventive routines are as important a part of your health maintenance as a good diet and exercise.

More and more Americans are beginning to turn to acupuncture. Before taking this step, however, most patients spend a lot of time and money on conventional treatments. When they begin to respond to acupuncture treatment, most new patients ask themselves why they had to suffer so long, why they had to endure poor health for so many years.

Insurance companies do not currently reimburse payment for nonphysician acupuncture treatment, so patients would not continue treatment if it didn't work. Some of my patients have returned for many years, long enough to have become old friends. Obviously, acupuncture pays off.

Most of the people attracted to this medical alternative think along these lines: "I want to avoid becoming dependent on drugs." "I am unhappy with the impersonal and costly care I have been subjected to, with no real benefit. Most doctors service illness and don't promote health." "I mistrust prescription drugs and their side effects."

If you recognize that your health is an ongoing process in which your total body well-being is paramount, you should promptly find a competent acupuncture practitioner.

Acupuncture is here to stay. It has survived and evolved for four thousand years and will continue to develop. It has a bright future in the United States as more and more positive clinical and research data emerge from our own and foreign medical centers. The time will soon come when acupuncture is routinely available all over the country. In the meantime, you can do no better than to take advantage of this wonderful resource now.

NOTES

1. Robert S. Mendelsohn, *Male Practice, How Doctors Manipulate Women.* Chicago: Contemporary Books, 1981, 7.
2. Arabella Melville and Colin Johnson, *Cured to Death.* New York: Stein and Day, 1982, 100.
3. "Script." 561, 1981. 12.
4. H. Jick, O. S. Miettenin, S. Shapiro, G. P. Lewis, V. Siskind and D. Slone. "Comprehensive Drug Surveillance." *Journal of the American Medical Association.* (2130): 1455, 1970.
5. E. W. Martin. Opening statement, DIA/AMA/FDA/PMA joint symposium, "Drug Information for Patients." *Drug Information Journal.* (11, Special Supplement) 1977, 2s-3s.
6. David Makofsky, "Malpractice and Medicine." *Where Medicine Fails,* 3rd ed. Brunswick, New Jersey: Transaction Books, 1979, 261-263.

7. *British Medical Journal*, (Vol. 282), 1982.

8. Primitivo T. Cruz. "Five Years' Experience with Traditional Acupuncture in a Research Program Clinic in Upstate New York." *American Journal of Acupuncture*. 10 (3): 255-258, 1982.

9. Y. T. Junnila Seppo. "Acupuncture Superior to Piroxicam in the Treatment of Osteoarthrosis." *American Journal of Acupuncture*. 10 (4): 341-346, 1982.

10. Cardiovascular Research Group. "Acupuncture Treatment of Cardiovascular Disease Complicated with Hyperlipidemia." *Chinese Acupuncture and Moxibustion*. 2 (4): 10-11, 1982.

11. Z. Liu. "Effects of Acupuncture and Moxibustion on the High Density Lipoprotein Cholesterol in Simple Obesity." *Acupuncture Research*. 15 (3): 227-231, 1990.

12. Y. Chen. "Clinical Research on Treating Senile Dementia by Combining Acupuncture with Acu-point-Injection." *Acupuncture Electric*. 17 (2): 61-73, 1992.

13. Hideharu Sakamoto. "Effect of Moxibustion on Aged Rats (Report IV): Reversal from Movement Disorders and Recovering Estrus Cycles." *Journal of Japan Society of Acupuncture*. 38 (2): 201 (31), 1988.

14. N. Shimura, et al. "Inhibitory Effects of Acupuncture, DPA and CMC on Sarcoma-180." *Journal of the Japan Society of Acupuncture and Moxibustion*. 31 (2): 122-126, 1981.

15. N. Shimura, et al. "Inhibition of Mouse Sarcoma by Acupuncture and D-phenylalanine." *Journal of Dental Research*. 61 (April): 598, 1982.

Appendix

ACUPUNCTURE RESOURCE DIRECTORY

I. ASSOCIATIONS

AAAOM (American Association of Acupuncture and Oriental Medicine). 50 Maple Place, Manhasset, New York 11030. Telephone: (202) 265-2287.

APAC (Acupuncture Political Action Committee). P.O. Box 155, Hollywood, California 90028.

International Veterinary Acupuncture Society. Department of Laboratory Animals Medicine, ML-571, College of Medicine, R-351, University of Cincinnati, Cincinnati, Ohio 45267.

The International Veterinary Acupuncture Society, c/o Meredith L. Snader, Executive Secretary. RD #1, Chester Springs, Pennsylvania 19425.

National Commission for Certification of Acupuncturists. 3952 North Southport, Chicago, Illinois 60613.

Traditional Acupuncture Foundation. American City Building, Suite 100, Columbia, Maryland 21044.

II. DETOX RESOURCE INFORMATION

An excellent source for all kinds of detox programs is the National Acupuncture Detoxification Association, 3115 Broadway, Rm. #51, New York, New York 10027.

For information specifically on alcohol rehabilitation, consult Ms. Patricia Colliton. Hennipin County Hospital, Minneapolis, Minnesota. She can be reached by calling (612) 559-4249.

For information on detox programs throughout New Mexico, you can talk with Nadine Bouleberri in Albuquerque at (505) 262-1801.

III. PUBLICATIONS

Acupuncture News and *International Journal of Chinese Medicine,* Center for Chinese Medicine, 230 South Garfield Avenue Monterey Park, California 91754.

American Acupuncturist, published by AAAOM, 50 Maple Place, Manhasset, New York 11030

American Journal of Acupuncture, 1400 Lost Acre Drive, Felton, California 95018.

Journal of Chinese Medicine, 68 Prince Edward's Road, Lewes, Sussex, England BN7-IBN.

Journal of Traditional Acupuncture, American City Building, Suite 100, Columbia, Maryland 21044.

SELECTED BIBLIOGRAPHY

Altman, Sheldon, D.M.V. *An Introduction to Acupuncture for Animals.* 1981. Chan's Corporation, P.O. Box 478, Monterey Park, California 91754.

Baldry, P. E. *Acupuncture Trigger Points and Musculoskeletal Pain.* 1989. London: Churchill Livingstone.

Barefoot Doctor's Manual. Revised ed., 1985. New York: Gramercy Publishing Co.

Berman, Edgar. *The Solid Gold Stethoscope.* 1976. New York: MacMillan.

Carlson, Ric. *The End of Medicine.* 1975. New York: Wiley.

Chaitow, Leon. *The Acupuncture Treatment of Pain.* 2nd ed. 1983. New York: Thorsons Publishers.

Chen, Jirui, M.D., and Nissi, Wang, eds. *Acupuncture Case Histories from China.* 1988. Seattle: Eastland Press.

Cheung, C. S., Yat Ki Li, C. A., and Vaik Kaw. *Mental Dysfunction as Treated by Traditional Chinese Medicine.* 1981. San Francisco: Traditional Chinese Medicine Publishers.

Dai-zhao, Zhang. *The Treatment of Cancer by Integrated Chinese-Western Medicine.* 1989. Boulder, Colorado: Blue Poppy Press.

Developments in Acupuncture Research. 1981. Beijing: People's Republic of China, Beijing.

Essentials of Chinese Acupuncture. 1980. Beijing: Foreign Language Press.

Flaws, Bob. *Free and Easy: Traditional Chinese Gynecology for American Women*. 1986. Boulder, Colorado: Blue Poppy Press.

Flaws, Bob. *Hit Medicine, Chinese Medicine Injury Management*. 1983. Boulder, Colorado: Blue Poppy Press.

Flaws, Bob. *Paths of Pregnancy*. 1983. Brookline, Massachusetts: Paradigm Publishers.

Flaws, Bob. *Turtle Tail and Other Tender Mercies: Traditional Chinese Pediatrics*. 1985. Boulder, Colorado: Blue Poppy Press.

Hammer, Leon. *Dragon Rises—Red Bird Flies: Psychology and Chinese Medicine*. 1990. Tarrytown, New York: Station Hill Press.

Hong-yen, Hsu, and Peacher, William G., eds. *Chinese Herbal Medicine and Therapy*. Revised ed. 1982. Los Angeles: Oriental Healing Arts Institute.

Hong-yen, Hsu, and Su-yen, Wang. *The Theory of Febrile Diseases and Its Clinical Applications*. 1982. Los Angeles: Oriental Healing Arts Institute.

Jayasuria, Anton. "A Scientific Review of Acupuncture" 1981. Paper read at the Seventh World Congress, Sri Lanka.

Kaptchuck, Ted. *The Web That Has No Weaver*. 1983. New York: Congdon and Weed.

Kinoshia, H. *Neuropathy*. 1968. Modern Acupuncture and Moxibustion Series. Kanagawa, Japan: Ido-no-nippon-sha.

Klide, Alan M. and Kung, H. Shui. *Veterinary Acupuncture*. 1977. Philadelphia: University of Pennsylvania Press.

Kurashima, S. *Circulatory, Renal, and Skin Diseases*. 1968. Modern Acupuncture and Moxibustion Series. Kanagawa, Japan: Ido-no-nippon-sha.

Larre, Claude, and Rochat de la Vallee, Elizabeth. *The Kidney. The Lungs. Chinese Medicine from the Classics*. 1989. The International Register of Oriental Medicine, Ricci Institute. Cambridge, England: Monthly Press.

Lewith, George T. *Acupuncture: Its Place in Western Medical Science*. 1982. Northhampshire, England: Thorsons Publishers.

Lewith, George T. *Acupuncture Treatment of Internal Disease*. 1985. New York: Thorsons Publishers.

Lewith, George T., and Lewith, M. R. *Modern Chinese Acupuncture*. Revised ed. 1983. New York: Thorsons Publishers.

Livingston, Martha, and Lowinger, P. *The Minds of the Chinese People: Mental Health in the New China*. 1983. Englewood-Cliffs, New

Jersey: Prentice-Hall

Low, Royston. *The Secondary Vessels of Acupuncture.* New York: Thorsons Publishers.

Low, Royston, and Turner, Roger N. *The Principles and Practice of Moxibustion.* 1981. Northhampshire, England: Thorsons Publishers.

Maciocai, Giovanni. *The Foundations of Chinese Medicine.* 1989. London: Churchill Livingstone.

Mann, Felix. *Acupuncture: The Ancient Art of Chinese Healing and How It Works Scientifically.* Revised ed. 1973. New York: Vintage Books.

Mann, Felix. *The Meridians of Acupuncture.* 1981. London: William Heinemann Medical Books.

Mao, T. T. *Quotations of Mao Tse-Tung,* Peking's People's Press, vol. 3 1953.

Melville, Arabella, and Johnson, Colin. *Cured to Death.* 1983. New York: Stein and Day.

Mendelsohn, Robert S. *Male Practice, How Doctors Manipulate Women.* 1981. Chicago: Contemporary Books.

Mori, H. *Disease of the Locomotor Apparatus.* 1968. Modern Acupuncture and Moxibustion Series. Kanagawa, Japan: Ido-no-nippon-sha.

O'Connor, John, and Bensky, Dan, trans. and eds. *Acupuncture: A Comprehensive Text.* 1981. Shanghai College of Traditional Medicine. Chicago: Eastland Press.

Omura, Yoshiaki. *Acupuncture Medicine.* 1982. Tokyo: Japan Publications.

Pomeranz, Bruce, and Stux, Gabriel. *Scientific Basis of Acupuncture.* 1988. Berlin: Springer-Verlag.

Porkett, Manfred. *The Theoretical Foundations of Chinese Medicine.* 1978. Cambridge, Massachusetts: MIT Press.

Porkett, Manfred, and Ullmann, Christian. *Chinese Medicine: Its History, Philosophy and Practice and Why It May One Day Dominate Medicine of the West.* 1982. New York: William Morow and Co.

Quinn, Joseph R., ed. *Medicine and Public Health in the People's Republic of China.* 1973. Washington, D.C.: Department of Health, Education and Welfare.

Requena, Yves. *Character and Health: The Relationship of Acupuncture and Psychology.* 1989. Brookline, Massachusetts: Paradigm

Publications.

Robinson, Nicola, and Berman, Monty. *Acupuncture in General Practice.* 1984. London: East Asia Co.

Scott, Julian. *The Treatment of Children by Acupuncture.* 1986. Sussex, England: Journal of Chinese Medicine.

So, James Tin Yau. *The Book of Acupuncture Points.* vol. I. 1984. Brookline, Massachusetts: Paradigm Publications.

St. John, Jeanne. "Acupressure Therapy in a School Environment for Handicapped Children." *American Journal of Acupuncture.* 15 (3): 227-238, 1987.

Strauss, Anselm L., ed. *Where Medicine Fails.* 3rd ed. 1979. New Brunswick, New Jersey: Transaction Books.

Tian-you, Feng. *Treatment of Soft Tissue Injury with Traditional Chinese and Western Medicine.* 1983. Beijing: People's Medical Publishing House.

Treating Deaf Mutes. 1972. Beijing: Foreign Language Press.

Unschuld, Paul V. *Forgotten Traditions of Ancient Chinese Medicine.* 1990. Brookline, Massachusetts: Paradigm Publications.

Veith, Ilza. *The Yellow Emperor's Classic of Internal Medicine.* New ed. 1972. Berkeley: University of California Press.

Wexu, Mario. *The Ear: Gateway to Balancing the Body.* 1982. New York: ASI Publishing Co.

Yoneyama, H. *Infantile Disease.* 1971. Modern Acupuncture and Moxibustion Series. Tobe Yokosuka, Japan: Soshichirotobe.

Youbang Chen and Laingyue Deng, eds. *Essentials of Contemporary Chinese Acupuncturists' Clinical Experience.* 1989. Beijing: Foreign Language Press.

Zhejiang College of Traditional Chinese Medicine. *A Handbook of Traditional Chinese Gynecology.* 1987. Boulder, Colorado: Blue Poppy Press.

INDEX

ABOUT THE AUTHOR

MARIE CARGILL is a Licensed Acupuncturist in the Boston area. She lectures at the New England School of Acupuncture and has had a private practice for more than a decade. Her pioneering work with animals has earned her international recognition. She is currently preparing a book on the use of acupuncture in gynecology and obstetrics.